Parkinson's Disease
Theory and Practice for Nurses

Parkinson's Disease

Theory and Practice for Nurses

Edited by

Lesley Swinn

Parkinson's Disease Nurse Specialist,
The National Hospital for Neurology
and Neurosurgery, University College
London Hospitals NHS Foundation Trust, London

W

WHURR PUBLISHERS
LONDON AND PHILADELPHIA

First published 2005
by Whurr Publishers Ltd
19b Compton Terrace
London N1 2UN England and
325 Chestnut Street, Philadelphia PA 19106 USA

British Library Cataloguing in Publication Data

A catalogue record for this book
is available from the British Library.

ISBN 1 86156 358 2

Typeset by Adrian McLaughlin, a@microguides.net
Printed and bound in the UK by Athenæum Press Ltd, Gateshead, Tyne & Wear.

Contents

Preface

This book was primarily written for nurses, but I hope that other health-care professionals will also find it useful and of value when they become involved in the care of people with Parkinson's disease (PD).

The aim of this book is to help the reader gain a better understanding of PD, its management and to gain insight into the many problems that people with PD and their families face on a daily basis. I hope that the book will equip the reader with the necessary knowledge and skills so that they are able to meet the ever-changing needs of people with PD.

All of the authors who contributed to this book have a wealth of experience and knowledge in caring for people with PD and most are recognized at a national and international level for their expertise. I would like to thank all of them for their valuable input and for managing to produce their chapters despite very busy full-time jobs.

Finally I would also like to thank my husband, Michael, for his advice, patience and encouragement.

Lesley Swinn
October 2004

The Contributors

Tess Astbury, Progressive supranuclear palsy Nurse Specialist, Progressive Supranuclear Palsy Association.

Catherine Best, Autonomic Nurse Specialist at The National Hospital for Neurology & Neurosurgery, London.

Ellie Borrell, Parkinson's disease Nurse Specialist at St Mary's Hospital, London.

Barbara Cormie, Information Resources Manager, Parkinson's Disease Society, London.

Ranan Dasgupta, Specialist Registrar in Urology formerly at The National Hospital for Neurology & Neurosurgery, London.

Peter Hagell, Senior Lecturer at the Department of Nursing, Lund University, Sweden.

Jacqui Handley, Parkinson's disease Nurse Specialist at Dorset County Hospital, Dorchester.

Collette Haslam, Uro-neurology clinical Nurse Specialist at The National Hospital for Neurology & Neurosurgery, London.

Gabrielle Irwin, Specialist Speech and Language Therapist at West Suffolk Hospital, Bury St Edmunds.

Carole Joint, Movement disorder Nurse Specialist at Radcliffe Infirmary, Oxford.

Carolyn Noble, Parkinson's disease Nurse Specialist at Greater Peterborough Primary Care Partnership, Peterborough.

Maggie Rose, Progressive supranuclear palsy Nurse Specialist, Progressive Supranuclear Palsy Association.

Lesley Swinn, Parkinson's disease Nurse Specialist at The National Hospital for Neurology & Neurosurgery, London.

Kirsten Turner, Parkinson's disease Nurse Specialist and Lecturer/Practitioner at Harold Wood Hospital, Essex Neuroscience Unit and South Bank University.

Karen Vernon, Secretary of the PDNSA (2001–2003), Community Neurology Nurse Specialist.

CHAPTER ONE

Pathogenesis of Parkinson's disease

LESLEY SWINN

Parkinson's disease (PD) is a common neurological condition which was first described in detail by James Parkinson in 1817. Great leaps in the understanding of PD have been made over the last decade or so, but, despite this, the precise causes of PD remain far from clear. This chapter will briefly discuss the neurochemistry and the pathological hallmarks of the disease and will then go on to discuss the various aetiological factors implicated in its development.

Review of normal motor function

Deep within the basal regions of the cerebral hemispheres of the brain lies a collection of nuclear masses called the basal ganglia. They consist of the globus pallidus, the putamen, the caudate nucleus, the subthalamic nucleus and the thalamus. The basal ganglia are crucial in the normal control of voluntary and involuntary movement.

The neurotransmitter dopamine (DA) is produced in the substantia nigra (SN) and this chemical influences the neuronal activity of the two main motor pathways within the basal ganglia circuit. One of the pathways has an excitatory effect (indirect pathway), whilst the other is inhibitory (direct pathway). The function of these pathways is to control the activity of the globus pallidus interna (GPi). The GPi has inhibitory connections to the thalamus and the thalamus, in turn, has excitatory connections to the motor cortex which facilitate movement. Dopamine increases the inhibitory activity of the direct pathway and decreases the excitatory activity of the indirect pathway. The net effect is to reduce the inhibitory activity of the GPi and thus allow the thalamus to facilitate movement. A simple schematic representation of the motor control is illustrated in Figure 1.1.

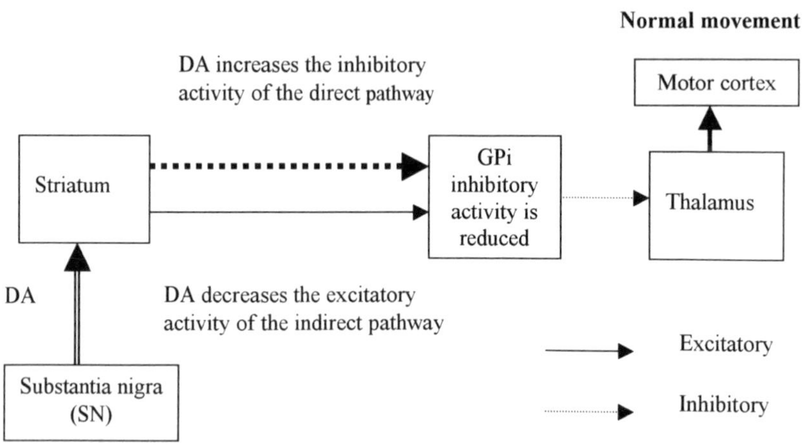

Figure 1.1 Normal motor control.

Parkinson's disease

Parkinson's disease occurs when the DA-containing (dopaminergic) cells within the SN progressively degenerate and die. The progressive loss of the dopaminergic (DA-ergic) cells results in the depletion of the neurotransmitter DA. Altered activity in other neurotransmitters has also been demonstrated in PD but the DA-ergic system is affected disproportionately by the neurodegenerative process.

The progressive loss of DA in PD results in an imbalance of activity between the direct and the indirect motor pathways within the basal ganglia motor circuit; there is an increase in excitatory activity within the indirect pathway and reduced inhibitory activity within the direct pathway. The net effect of this is to increase GPi activity, which consequently inhibits the thalamocortical outflow so movement is inhibited (Lang and Lozano 1998a, 1998b). A simple schematic representation of the activity within the basal ganglia motor circuit caused by PD is illustrated in Figure 1.2.

The nigrostriatal neurons have a high degree of plasticity and the symptoms of PD do not become evident until there is about 50–70% DA-ergic cell loss (Hornykiewicz 1975, Riederer and Wuketich 1976). There are two compensatory mechanisms which account for the high degree of plasticity. First, there is a marked increase in the DA turnover in the remaining nigrostriatal neurons and second, the postsynaptic DA receptors become supersensitive. Unfortunately, these compensatory mechanisms eventually fail and this leads to the emergence of symptoms.

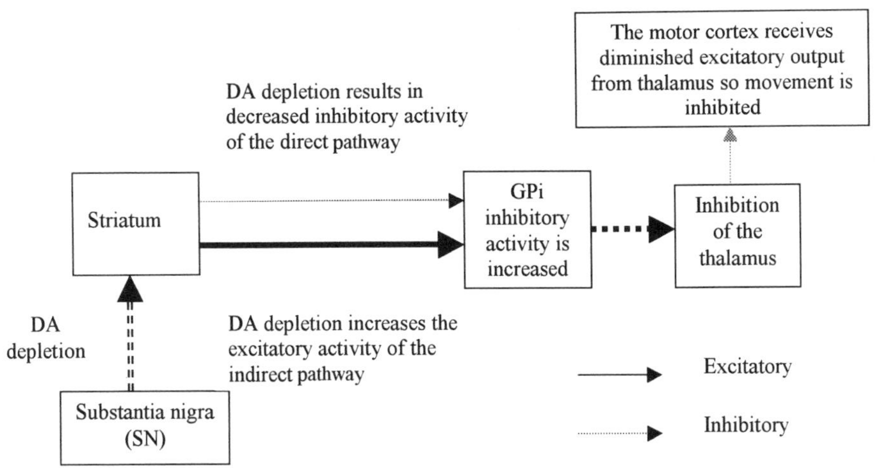

Figure 1.2 Parkinson's disease and the basal ganglia.

Pathology of Parkinson's disease

The two pathological hallmarks of PD are DA-ergic neuronal loss within the SN and the presence of Lewy bodies. Neuronal loss is not isolated to the SN but occurs in other areas of the brain such as the hypothalamus, sympathetic ganglia and the mesolimbic and mesocortical DA-ergic neurons (Bethlem and den Hartog Jager 1960; Gibb and Lees 1988).

Lewy bodies are neuronal inclusions which are found in the areas of neuronal degeneration. They are not specific to PD as they are also found in other neurological conditions, including cortical basal degeneration, progressive supranuclear palsy and motor neurone disease (Gibb and Lees 1988), but the distribution of the Lewy body is specific to PD. The exact purpose of the Lewy body is still unclear but one possible function is that it might aid elimination of damaged proteins from cells (Lowe 1994).

Aetiology of Parkinson's disease

An increasing body of evidence now indicates that PD may arise from a variety of insults causing damage or death of the DA neurons. These include the ageing process, genetic susceptibility, oxidative stress and environmental toxins (Riederer and Lange 1992).

The ageing process

Advancing age is the single most important risk factor for developing PD

(Stewart 2001). Epidemiological studies demonstrate an exponential increase in the incidence of PD with increasing age. The prevalence varies from 0.1% in the general population to 2% in people over the age of 80 years (Mutch et al 1986). The exact role of the ageing process in PD is unclear, but a number of pathological changes are similar in both PD and the normal ageing process, including a decrease in the number of pigmented neurons within the SN (McGeer et al 1977) and a decrease in striatal DA (Kish et al 1992). However, the distribution of the neuronal cell loss in the ageing brain is different from that seen in PD.

Genetics of Parkinson's disease

The vast majority of causes of PD are sporadic, but family history is the next most important risk factor after age. In the last few years several genes have been identified as rare causes of PD.

Park 1

Park 1 was the first gene to be identified and was found within a large Italian family (known as the Contursi kindred). The gene is located on chromosome 4q (Polymeropoulos et al 1997) and codes for a small protein called alpha-synuclein. Alpha-synuclein has been found to be a major component of the Lewy body (Spillantini et al 1997). It is likely that the accumulation of alpha-synuclein within the Lewy body is central to the development of PD (Olanow and Tatton 1999). However, gene mutations of this protein have not been found in sporadic PD.

Park 1 is inherited in an autosomal dominant fashion but it is extremely rare and has been found in only a few other families throughout the world.

Park 2 (Parkin)

This gene, commonly known as Parkin, is inherited in an autosomal recessive fashion and has been mapped to chromosome 6q25 (Matsumine et al 1997). Mutations of this gene cause an enzyme called ubiquitin protein ligase to lose its activity. This enzyme is thought to be involved with the degradation of abnormal proteins. Postmortem studies have demonstrated degeneration of the SN, but unlike idiopathic disease, Lewy bodies are not present (Mori et al 1998). Patients with this gene predominantly have juvenile onset disease. This gene has been found to be responsible for 77% of patients who developed PD with an age of onset of 20 years and younger but only 3% of patients with onset between 30 and 45 years (Lucking et al 2000).

Other genes

Other single gene defects have recently been discovered and searches for new genes continue. It is increasingly apparent that there are several genetically distinct forms of PD caused by different mutations in single genes.

However, it must be remembered that PD in the great majority of patients is sporadic and single gene defects do not account for most of these cases.

Environmental factors

A number of environmental factors seem to be associated with an increased risk of developing PD; these include exposure to agricultural and industrial chemicals, and rural living. A number of specific toxins have been associated with the development of parkinsonism but no specific toxin has been found in the brain of PD patients; the parkinsonism associated with these toxins is not typical of idiopathic PD (Olanow and Tatton 1999). The strongest evidence supporting the environmental hypothesis relates to the toxin 1,2,3,6-methyl-phenyl-tetrahydropyridine (MPTP). MPTP is a by-product of a meperidine analogue, an illicit drug that was sold as an injectable narcotic in California in the late 1970s. Some of the drug addicts who repeatedly injected this drug rapidly developed an akinetic-rigid syndrome that resembled PD both clinically and pathologically (Langston et al 1983). It is now known that this toxin causes DA-ergic cell death mainly through free-radical formation and inhibition of ATP synthesis. Although MPTP is a rare cause of parkinsonism, its discovery led to an enormous leap in the understanding of PD as it provided researchers with an excellent animal model. However, to date, no other MPTP-like factor has been identified (Olanow and Tatton 1999).

Gene–environment interaction

An increasing number of studies are now suggesting that genetic susceptibility to PD, mediated by deficient enzyme systems involved in the disposal of neurotoxins, may explain a role for both genes and the environment in the development of the disease (Foltynie et al 2002). Inheritance of certain genes may lead to the development of the disease, whereas other genes may require exposure to environmental agents before the disease can evolve.

Mechanism of dopamine neuronal loss

It is thought that programmed cell death (apoptosis) is responsible for the DA-ergic neuronal loss found in PD. A number of factors have been implicated in the process of apoptotic cell death of the SN, including oxidative stress, mitochondrial dysfunction and excitotoxicity.

Oxidative stress

Mounting evidence points to the formation of free radicals as a key precursor to DA-ergic cell loss. Excessive free-radical production is known to result in lipid peroxidation causing membrane damage and neuronal death (Riederer and Lange 1992). Postmortem studies have demonstrated that oxidative stress takes place in the SN of patients with PD. It remains unknown whether there is an excessive formation of free radicals in PD through oxidative degradation of DA, and/or whether there is a reduction in the scavenging systems which normally prevent the accumulation of free radicals.

Mitochondrial dysfunction

Brain studies have shown that mitochondrial dysfunction occurs in PD. Studies have found a selective decrease in complex 1 activity of the mitochondrial respiratory chain in the cells within the SN of PD patients (Schapira et al 1989). It remains to be established whether the complex 1 deficiency is attributable to the presence of neurotoxins or is genetically determined (Foltynie et al 2002). Olanow and Tatton (1999) have postulated that the complex 1 deficit might contribute to neuronal vulnerability and lead to apoptosis.

Excitotoxicity

Excessive excitatory activity can result in cell damage (excitotoxicity). The reduction in energy metabolism due to mitochondrial dysfunction may result in increased glutamate activity. Glutamate is an excitatory neurotransmitter and the SN is rich in glutamate receptors. Excessive glutamate activity can result in disproportionate calcium influx into the cell and this, in turn, causes excitotoxicity and cell damage.

Conclusion

The cause of PD remains unknown but there is accumulating evidence which suggests that PD arises from multiple aetiologies rather than one single factor. Evidence also suggests that several overlapping factors are implicated in the process of cell death. A schematic representation of the factors implicated in the pathogenesis of PD is shown in Figure 1.3. It is hoped that greater understanding of the aetiology and pathogenesis of PD in the future will ultimately lead to the development of effective neuroprotective agents that can slow the rate of the neuronal loss.

Key points

- Parkinson's disease (PD) is a common neurological condition caused by the progressive loss of the neurotransmitter dopamine.

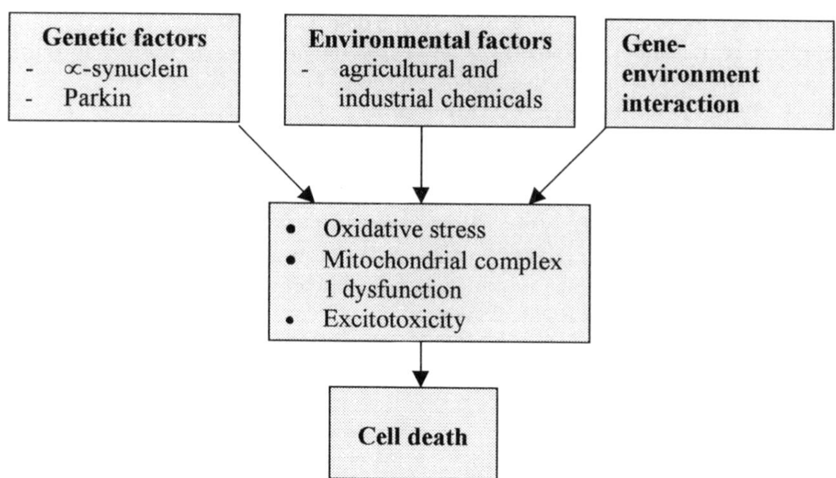

Figure 1.3 Factors implicated in the pathogenesis of Parkinson's disease. (Adapted from Stewart 2001)

- Depleted levels of dopamine result in an imbalance within the basal ganglia motor circuitry.
- The cause of PD remains unknown but it is likely to be caused by multiple aetiologies rather than one single factor.
- A number of factors are implicated in the process of neuronal loss including oxidative stress, mitochondrial dysfunction and excitotoxicity.

References

Bethlem J and den Hartog Jager W A (1960) The incidence and characteristics of Lewy bodies in idiopathic paralysis agitans (Parkinson's disease). Journal of Neurology, Neurosurgery and Psychiatry 23: 74–80.

Foltynie T, Sawcer S, Brayne C and Barker R A (2002) The genetic basis of Parkinson's disease. Journal of Neurology, Neurosurgery and Psychiatry 73: 363–370.

Gibb W R G and Lees A J (1988) The relevance of the Lewy body to the pathogenesis of idiopathic Parkinson's disease. Journal of Neurology, Neurosurgery and Psychiatry 5(1): 745–752.

Hornykiewicz O (1975) Parkinson's disease and its chemotherapy. Biochemical Pharmocology 24: 1061–1065.

Kish S L, Shannak K, Rajput A et al (1992) Aging produces a specific pattern of striatal dopamine loss: implications for the etiology of idiopathic Parkinson's disease. Journal of Neurochemistry 58: 642–648.

Lang A E and Lozano A M (1998a) Medical progress: Parkinson's disease. First of two parts. New England Journal of Medicine 339: 1044–1053.

Lang A E and Lozano A M (1998b) Medical progress: Parkinson's disease. Second of two parts. New England Journal of Medicine 339: 1130–1143.

Langston J W, Ballard P A, Tetrud J W et al (1983) Chronic parkinsonism in humans due to a product of meperidine analog synthesis. Science 219: 979–980.

Lowe J (1994) Lewy bodies. In: D B Calne (ed.) Neurodegenerative Diseases. Philadelphia: WB Saunders pp. 51–69.

Lucking C B, Durr A, Bonifati V et al (2000) Association between early onset Parkinson's disease and mutations in the parkin gene. New England Journal of Medicine 342: 1560–1567.

Matsumine H, Saito M, Shimoda M S et al (1997) Localization of a gene for autosomal recessive form of juvenile parkinsonism to chromosome 6q25.2-27. American Journal of Human Genetics 60: 588–596.

McGeer P L, McGeer E G, Suzuki J S (1977) Aging and the extrapyramidal function. Archives of Neurology 34: 44–45.

Mori H, Kondo T, Yokochi M et al (1998) Pathologic and biochemical studies of juvenile parkinsonism linked to chromosome 6q. Neurology 51: 890–892.

Mutch W J, Dingwall-Fordyce I, Downie A W et al (1986) Parkinson's disease in a Scottish city. British Medical Journal 292: 534–536.

Olanow C W and Tatton W G (1999) Etiology and pathogenesis of Parkinson's disease. Annual Review of Neuroscience 22: 123–144.

Parkinson J (1817) An Essay on the Shaking Palsy. First published London: Sherwood, Neely and Jones. Modern edition: London Macmillan Magazines and Parkinson's Disease Society of the United Kingdom (1992).

Polymeropoulos M H, Higgins J J, Golbe L I et al (1996) Mapping a gene for Parkinson's disease to chromosome 4q21-q23. Science 276: 2045–2047.

Riederer P and Lange K W (1992) Pathogenesis of Parkinson's disease. Annals of Neurology 35(5): 586–591.

Riederer P and Wuketich S (1976) Time course of nigrostriatal degeneration in Parkinson's disease; a detailed study of influential factors in human brain analogues. Journal of Neural Transmission. Parkinson's Disease and Dementia Section 38: 277–301.

Schapira A H V, Cooper J M and Dexter D (1989) Mitochondrial complex 1 deficiency in Parkinson's disease. Annals of Neurology 26: 122–123.

Spillanti M G, Schmidt M L, Lee V M et al (1997) Alpha-synuclein in Lewy bodies (Letter). Nature 388: 839–840.

Stewart D A (2001) Pathology, aetiology and pathogenesis. In: J R Player and J V Hindle (eds.) Parkinson's Disease in the Older Patient. London: Arnold pp. 11–29.

CHAPTER TWO
Diagnosing Parkinson's disease

PETER HAGELL AND LESLEY SWINN

In its classical presentation, Parkinson's disease (PD) is often regarded a generally easy condition to diagnose. Indeed, this is one of the few disorders that, in principle, can be identified by a mere quick glance at an affected individual walking down the street. However, this is not always the case. Autopsy-based studies have shown that, even among neurologists, diagnostic accuracy is imperfect, with up to about 25% of cases carrying an erroneous diagnosis of PD at the time of death (Rajput et al 1991; Hughes et al 1992). There are currently no biological markers available that will lead to a completely definite diagnosis of PD during life and the diagnosis remains entirely clinical. This chapter will discuss the clinical symptoms of PD and will cover issues relating to diagnosing PD. It will also highlight the importance of patient education and support at the time of diagnosis. While an exhaustive coverage of all aspects of the diagnosis of PD is beyond the scope of this chapter, relevant references are included to guide the interested reader to more specific literature.

Epidemiology of Parkinson's disease

Parkinson's disease is a relatively common chronically progressive neurodegenerative disorder, affecting a significant minority of the population. In various European studies during the past decade (Tandberg et al 1995; Fall et al 1996; Wermuth et al 1997; Errea et al 1999; Kuopio et al 1999; Vines et al. 1999; Schrag et al 2000; Wermuth et al 2000; Taba and Asser 2002, 2003), its age-adjusted prevalence has varied between 76 and 183 cases per 100,000, with an annual incidence of between 7 and 17 new cases per 100,000 persons. In a recent community-based UK cross-sectional epidemiological study (carried out in the London area) Schrag and collaborators estimated the crude and age-adjusted prevalence of PD to be 128 and 168 per 100,000, respectively (Schrag et al 2000). While PD may occur at any age, it is rare before the age of 30 years; thereafter there is a progressive and expotential age-related rise in incidence, and the prevalence in the 80+ age group has been estimated to be between 1 and 4%. The mean age of onset is around 60 years (Quinn 1997). Most studies have found a slight excess of male to female cases.

Clinical features of Parkinson's disease

Parkinson's disease is a clinicopathological condition which is characterized by parkinsonism caused by neuronal loss, with the presence of Lewy bodies, within the substantia nigra (Gibb and Lees 1988). These neurons project to the striatum where they release the transmitter dopamine (DA) and their degeneration thus causes a striatal DA deficiency. The pathology of PD involves numerous areas and transmitter systems, but the clinical implications of these alterations are poorly understood. The striatal DA deficiency, secondary to degeneration of nigrostriatal DA-ergic neurons, is believed to be the underlying cause of the majority of the motor manifestations of PD.

The nigrostriatal neurons have a high degree of plasticity and the symptoms of PD do not become evident until there is about 50–70% DA-ergic cell loss (Hornykiewicz 1975; Riederer and Wuketich 1976). The onset of symptoms is usually insidious. The disease usually presents with unilateral symptoms that eventually progress to bilateral involvement, although the side of symptom onset usually remains the more severely affected throughout the course of the disease (Poewe and Wenning 1998). PD is characterized by four main neurological features: paucity of movement, rigidity, tremor and postural instability.

Paucity of movement

This is the most characteristic motor symptom of basal ganglia dysfunction in PD (Vingerhoets et al 1997) and is also one of the most disabling features of the disease (Lyons et al 1997). The paucity of movement in PD consists of slowness of initiation of movement with progressive reduction in speed and amplitude of repeated movements (Sawle 1999). It therefore consists of three main entities: bradykinesia (slowness of movement), hypokinesia (reduced movement) and akinesia (inability to initiate movement) (Marsden 1989; Macphee 2001). These terms are often used interchangeably, and here we will mainly use the term bradykinesia. Many of the clinical characteristics of PD, such as hypomimia, micrographia, dysphagia and respiratory difficulties, are, at least in part, various expressions of bradykinesia. Bradykinesia is a major cause of disability as it is responsible for the slowness that patients demonstrate in performing the simplest of tasks such as dressing, preparing meals, eating and bathing.

Rigidity

Rigidity is the increase in resistance to passive movements around a joint. The term 'lead-pipe' describes smooth resistance whereas 'cogwheeling' denotes rigidity that feels as though the joint is moving through teeth of a cog and is believed to occur due to superimposed or underlying tremor (Quinn 1995). Rigidity can affect any part of the body. The increase in muscle tone is evident throughout the range of movement upon passive flexion and extension; it tends to be more evident in flexors, which contributes to the classical flexed posture seen in PD. Rigidity is mainly to be considered a sign rather than a symptom; patients may notice a feeling of 'stiffness' to which rigidity may contribute, but the correlation between the two is generally poor and the latter is probably often mainly attributable to bradykinesia (Jankovic 1992).

Tremor

Tremor is seen in about 75% of patients with PD (Gelb et al 1999) and is the symptom that most often causes the patient to seek medical help. There are many types of tremor, such as postural tremor, action tremor and intention tremor, which can be related to specific brain lesions and/or dysfunctions. The tremor that is typical of PD occurs at rest and disappears or decreases with action. Rest tremor of the hands is often described as a 'pill-rolling' tremor because it looks as though a pill is being rolled between the thumb and the forefinger. The tremor in PD is fairly slow, around 4–6 Hz. The rest tremor of PD is usually most prominent in the hands and also appears in the lower extremities and the chin/jaws; it is rarely seen in the head (Sawle 1999). DA neuron loss in the substantia nigra is thought to be an underlying cause (Carr 2002), although tremor is poorly correlated with the striatal DA deficit (Vingerhoets et al 1997) and probably results from disruption of various components of the basal ganglia, as well as other related regions (e.g. the thalamus, cortex and cerebellum).

Postural instability

Postural instability is often included as one of the four core symptoms of PD but appears some time into the progression of disease and signifies the transition from mild to moderate PD, as defined by the Hoehn and Yahr (HY) staging of the disease (Hoehn and Yahr 1967). While perhaps the least specific, postural instability appears to be one of the most disabling of the four cardinal PD symptoms (Jankovic 1992; Lyons et al 1997) and may cause the patient to fall. Postural instability together with, for example, disturbances of gait and speech, may, at least in part, be the result of non-DA-ergic degenerations occurring with progressive disease (Bonnet et al 1987).

Non-motor features

The clinical presentation of PD goes well beyond that of neurological motor features. Although non-motor features are generally less well recognized and understood, to a certain extent some of them may be related to the primary motor disturbances. Non-motor features of PD include depression, neuropsychological dysfunctions, cognitive deficiencies with or without dementia, olfactory deficiency, sleep disturbance, fatigue, pain and other sensory phenomena, and various autonomic disturbances (e.g. hypotension, orthostasis, sweating dysfunction, and bowel, bladder and sexual dysfunctions) (Brown et al 1990; Cummings 1992; Edwards et al 1992; Jankovic 1992; Hawkes et al 1997; Ford 1998; Karlsen et al 1999; Sawle 1999; Glosser 2001; Shulman et al 2002; Swinn et al 2003).

Presenting symptoms

Presenting motor symptoms can vary considerably but common initial problems before the diagnosis is made may include:

- General slowness in most activities
- Tremor in a part of the body, typically either of the hands
- Handwriting becoming smaller (micrographia)
- Difficulty with walking

In some cases, it is not the patient who notices that something is wrong; often their partner or a close family member may notice more subtle changes such as loss of facial expression or reduced arm swing while walking. Frozen shoulder is thought to be a fairly common initial symptom caused by rigidity of the shoulder muscles, and it is not uncommon for patients to be referred to orthopaedic teams, with complaints of shoulder stiffness or pain, instead of neurology teams (Riley et al 1989).

A common early non-motor symptom is anosmia (loss of smell) which is thought to affect at least 70% of patients with PD (Doty et al 1988; Hawkes et al 1997). Other non-motor features that may be present before the onset of PD motor symptoms include depression and vegetative, sensory and neuropsychological symptoms and signs. However, none of these early non-motor features are well enough characterized to allow clinicians to link them to the diagnosis of PD in the absence of neurological motor deficits compatible with the disease.

Diagnosis

There are no biological markers to aid a definite diagnosis of PD, so it is diagnosed entirely on clinical grounds. Clearly this may result in a degree of misdiagnosis and this problem has been highlighted in two large brain bank series: only about 75% of cases carrying a diagnosis of PD at death met the established neuropathological criteria for idiopathic PD (Rajput et al 1991; Hughes et al 1992). This is a misdiagnosis rate of over 20%, but it is thought that the rate of misdiagnosis in the early stages by non-specialists is probably higher (Quinn 1995). As a result, various diagnostic criteria have been suggested to improve the accuracy of clinical diagnosis. Among these, the United Kingdom Parkinson's Disease Society Brain Bank diagnostic criteria (Gibb and Lees 1988), which are based on post-mortem histopathology, are now generally accepted as best clinical practice. These diagnostic criteria can be broken down into three clear steps:

- Establishment of the presence of a parkinsonian disorder
- Exclusion of other causes
- Presence of supportive criteria (Table 2.1)

Table 2.1 United Kingdom Parkinson's Disease Society Brain Bank clinical diagnostic criteria (Gibb and Lees 1988)

Step 1 Diagnosis of parkinsonian syndrome

1. Bradykinesia (slowness of initiation of voluntary movement with progressive reduction in speed and amplitude of repetitive actions)
2. AND at least one of the following:
    - Muscular rigidity
    - Rest tremor 4–6 Hz
    - Postural instability not caused by primary visual, vestibular, cerebellar or proprioceptive dysfunction

Step 2 Exclusion criteria for Parkinson's disease

History of repeated strokes with stepwise progression of parkinsonian features
History of repeated head injury
History of definite encephalitis
Oculogyric crises
Neuroleptic treatment at onset of symptoms
More than one affected relative
Sustained remission
Strictly unilateral features after 3 years
Supranuclear gaze palsy

Table 2.1 contd

Step 2 Exclusion criteria for Parkinson's disease (contd)

Cerebellar signs
Early severe autonomic involvement
Early severe dementia with disturbance of memory, language and praxis
Babinski sign
Presence of cerebal tumour or communicating hydrocephalus on CT scan
Negative response to large doses of levodopa (if malabsorption excluded)
Exposure to MPTP

Step 3 Supportive prospective positive criteria for Parkinson's disease (three or more required for diagnosis of definite Parkinson's disease)

Unilateral onset
Rest tremor present
Progressive disorder
Persistent asymmetry affecting side of onset most
Excellent response (70–100%) to levodopa
Severe levodopa-induced chorea
Levodopa response for 5 years or more
Clinical course of 10 years or more

Because none of the features included in the United Kingdom Parkinson's Disease Society Brain Bank diagnostic criteria is sufficiently specific and sensitive to diagnose the disease, Gelb et al (1999) have suggested various combinations of parameters to define the probability of the diagnosis. These are listed in Table 2.2.

Table 2.2 Levels of probability of the diagnosis of PD based on the United Kingdom Parkinson's Disease Society Brain Bank diagnostic criteria (abridged from Gelb et al 1999)

Possible PD	Presence of at least two cardinal symptoms (including bradykinesia or tremor) Absence of atypical symptoms Documented response to levodopa or DA agonist (or absence of adequate therapeutic trial)
Probable PD	Presence of at least three cardinal symptoms Absence of atypical symptoms for at least 3 years Documented substantial and sustained response to levodopa or DA agonist
Definite PD	Presence of all above criteria Autopsy confirmation

Applying rigorous criteria such as those outlined above certainly reduces misdiagnosis substantially (to <10%), in particular among specialists, but does not guarantee complete accuracy (Hughes et al 2001, 2002). Difficulties in diagnosis of PD can be evident especially in early disease, as symptoms and signs may be subtle and many of the core symptoms also occur in other conditions. The diagnosis is also difficult to make in older patients as the prevalence of other neurological manifestations (including PD differential diagnoses) increases with age and may blur the clinical picture (Macphee 2001).

Most patients will visit their general practitioner (GP) when they think something is amiss, and most GPs will refer patients to either a neurologist or geriatrician for an opinion and confirmation of a suspect case of PD. The first step in making the diagnosis is to take a full history from the patient. This will cover factors such as the time of onset, presenting symptoms, speed and pattern of progress, past and presently known disorders, substance exposure (pharmaceuticals and environmental/occupational) and a family history. The clinician will then conduct a physical examination that will show whether signs of PD (bradykinesia, tremor and/or rigidity) are present and whether the patient is experiencing any additional, atypical, features that may speak against the diagnosis of PD. Such atypical features include supranuclear gaze abnormalities, cerebellar or pyramidal signs and early onset of mental, autonomic or bulbar problems. An experienced movement disorder clinician may make the diagnosis straight away, especially if there are no unusual signs or symptoms, but it is not unusual for certain investigations to be carried out in order to exclude other causes that may explain the patient's complaints. Finally, or sometimes in parallel with such investigations (depending on the severity of the patient's complaints and disability), a therapeutic trial with levodopa or a DA agonist is initiated and the therapeutic response is evaluated as an important step in ascertaining the clinical diagnosis of PD. Although it may appear fairly straightforward, in practice the diagnosis of PD can be difficult, especially in differentiating possible PD from some other neurological disorders that can present with a clinical picture very similar or virtually identical to idiopathic PD, particularly early in their development. Indeed, the time course of the disease, in combination with DA-ergic response and symptomatic profile, is to be considered one of the most important factors for an accurate diagnosis (Gelb et al 1999; Lachenmayer 2003).

Differential diagnosis of PD

A common feature of all differential diagnoses of PD is that they present with a parkinsonian syndrome, i.e. parkinsonism. The term parkinsonism is an umbrella term describing any clinical condition (including PD) presenting with symptoms of bradykinesia, rigidity, tremor and/or postural instability (Marsden 1994). The number of conditions that can present with parkinsonism and thus constitute differential diagnoses of PD is vast, at least 50, and a review of them all is clearly beyond the scope of this chapter. However, a brief list of some of the more common differential diagnoses of PD is shown in Table 2.3. For a thorough review of these and other conditions that may mimic PD, the reader is referred to the references provided in Table 2.3.

Table 2.3 Common differential diagnoses of PD

Diagnosis	References*
Multiple system atrophy (MSA)	Gilman et al 1999; Gilman 2002
Progressive supranuclear palsy (PSP)	Litvan et al 1996; Tolosa et al 2002
Corticobasal degeneration	Riley and Lang 2000; Kumar et al 2002
Dementia with Lewy bodies	McKeith et al 1996; McKeith et al 2004
Drug-induced parkinsonism	Hubble 1997
Vascular parkinsonism	Yamanouchi and Nagura 1997; Winikates and Jankovic 1999
Essential tremor	Deuschl et al 1998; Pahwa and Lyons 2003

* Refers to published diagnostic criteria (where available) and thorough descriptions of the respective conditions. The reader is also referred to Litvan et al (2003) who provide an up-to-date review of available clinical diagnostic criteria for the main parkinsonian disorders. See also Chapters 12 and 13 of this volume for more information on PSP and MSA.

To alert the clinical practitioner that it may be wise to stop and think twice about the diagnosis of PD, a set of 'red flags' have been proposed (Table 2.4). These are not diagnostic, and some can be seen in idiopathic PD, but they constitute signs and symptoms that should raise suspicion about the diagnosis. As a general rule, the more flags that are present in one patient the more suspicious one should be about the diagnosis.

It is important for nurses and other clinical practitioners to be aware of signs that may indicate that the patient does not suffer from idiopathic PD. This is because the prognosis can be drastically different (worse) in other parkinsonian disorders, and inadequate treatment, for example increasing doses of DA-ergic drugs, may lead to additional problems in terms of adverse effects, while providing little or no additional benefit.

Table 2.4 Clinical 'red flags' (from Quinn 1995)

Early instability/falls	Blepharospasm
Rapid progression	Cold, dusky extremities
Poor/waning levodopa response	Contractures
Absent/atypical levodopa-induced dyskinesias	Disproportionate antecollis
Lower body parkinsonism	Severe dysphonia/dysarthria/dysphagia
Autonomic failure	Inspiratory sighs
Pyramidal signs	Pseudobulbar crying
Cerebellar signs	Palilalia/palilogia
Dementia	Groaning
Downgaze palsy	Respiratory stridor
Levator inhibition	Jerky tremor or myoclonus
'Wheelchair sign' (early permanent need of wheelchair)	

Diagnostic investigations

As stated earlier, there is currently no biomarker or any other test available that is completely specific for PD or the more common alternative diagnoses. However, various investigations and tests are often performed, either to exclude other causes of parkinsonism or to strengthen the suspect diagnosis (whether it is PD or another parkinsonian condition). Here we briefly review investigations that may be carried out to exclude other causes of parkinsonism. The list is not exhaustive but constitutes a selection of some of the more commonly used and available tests.

Structural neuroimaging

Computerized tomography (CT)

A CT scan does not reveal any PD-specific findings. However, it may be useful to rule out structural abnormalities such as hydrocephalus, space-occupying lesions, cerebral vascular accidents or other lesions that may give rise to parkinsonian features. Apart from such circumstances, CT scans are of no value for the diagnosis of PD.

Magnetic resonance imaging (MRI)

MRI may be useful for viewing structural changes or abnormalities within the basal ganglia. Specific changes on MRI have been described for several parkinsonian disorders (Savoiardo 2003; Yekhlef et al 2003). For example, studies have found atrophy of the substantia nigra in PD, and a decreased signal in the putamen of patients with poor response to DA-ergic drugs, in particular in those with the striatonigral degeneration variant of MSA. Standard MRI scans can provide important additional information in ambiguous cases, particularly if the scans demonstrate specific changes that favour an alternative diagnosis over PD. However, these changes may be absent in the early stages of the disease and their specificity and sensitivity (especially in early disease) are unclear, which might confound the problem of diagnosis.

Functional neuroimaging

Functional neuroimaging, such as SPECT and PET, may be requested if there is some doubt about the diagnosis. SPECT and PET provide in vivo information about regional changes in brain metabolism, blood flow, terminal function and receptor binding in PD by studying the uptake and distribution of various ligands. The specific function that needs to be studied will guide the choice of ligand; in PD there are specific ligands available for the study of, for example, both pre- and postsynaptic dopaminergic function in the striatum. In principle, both techniques can be used for essentially the same purposes, but SPECT is slightly less sensitive than PET. SPECT is, however, more widely available and less expensive than PET, which tends to make it more relevant from a clinical perspective. Studies have shown that both SPECT and PET investigations of DA terminal and striatal function can detect PD in the very early stages and can help distinguish atypical syndromes from PD with at least 80% specificity (Brooks 1998). SPECT and PET can provide valuable information in cases that cause diagnostic difficulties due to, for example, ambiguous clinical presentation or unequivocal response to levodopa. Furthermore, they may be of value to confirm a clinical diagnosis of PD. However, most experts agree that they should not be used routinely in clinical practice and the decision to perform functional brain imaging as part of the diagnostic workup of a parkinsonian patient should be made after careful consideration by an expert clinician (Dodel et al 2003; Poewe and Scherfler 2003).

Acute dopaminergic drug challenge

Acute pharmacological challenges, using either levodopa or apomorphine, were introduced during the 1980s (Barker et al 1989; Esteguy et al 1985). Clinical assessments are performed before and after each test dose of either levodopa or apomorphine and a response of 15–20% or more on either the motor examination section (section III) of the unified PD rating scale (UPDRS) (Fahn et al 1987) or the timed hand/arm movement (HAM) test (Defer et al 1999; Hagell 2000) is regarded a positive dopaminergic response (Gasser et al 1992; van Hilten et al 1997; Rossi et al 2000) (see also Chapter 5 for a detailed description of the apomorphine test).

Since their introduction, acute dopaminergic drug challenges have become quite common. However, there has been much debate on the clinical accuracy or use of these acute drug challenge tests in the diagnostic workup of parkinsonian patients; some argue that they have 'reasonable precision' (Hughes et al 1990) and recommend their use (Pogarell and Oertel 1999), whereas others recommend against using them as a diagnostic tool (Bhatia et al 1998; Hughes 1999; Clarke and Davies 2000). Their proposed role in diagnosing PD was based on the assumption that most patients with PD respond well to dopaminergic drugs, whereas those with other parkinsonian syndromes do not. A positive drug challenge, even very early in the disease, was thus presumed to predict a diagnosis of PD. However, up to about 50% of patients with MSA and 20% of PSP patients show an initial response to dopaminergic drugs. In MSA, this response may continue in late stages of the disease in up to 20% of patients. Furthermore, there is a small fraction of patients with pathologically proved PD who fail to respond. Hence, while dopaminergic responsiveness is an important diagnostic criterion for PD, on its own it is not necessarily a good discriminator between idiopathic PD and other parkinsonian conditions in early stages of disease. However, this does not mean that acute dopaminergic drug challenges do not have a role in the clinical management of PD (Hughes 1999; Albanese et al 2001). The apomorphine test has, for example, been suggested as a useful tool to guide what motor response might be obtained with higher doses of levodopa, to assess the dopaminergic responsiveness of specific features of the disease, or to reassess cases where the response to a long trial of oral DA-ergic medication has had little, no or equivocal effects (Hughes 1999; Albanese et al 2001).

Miscellaneous tests

In addition to the tests outlined above, there are a number of other investigations that may be of relevance in the individual patient. These include, for example, various autonomic and neurophysiological tests, and, in the future, genetic testing may become more common. However, it is beyond the scope of this chapter to review these in any detail and the interested reader is referred to relevant specific literature (Valls-Sole 2000; Bonifati et al 2001; Goldstein 2003; Litvan et al 2003; Micieli et al 2003).

The impact of diagnosis on the patient

Most patients will remember the exact moment when they are given the diagnosis of PD; for some it will not be unexpected but for others it will be a bombshell out of the blue. Patients' reactions will vary greatly but feelings such as horror, fear, isolation, guilt, anger and injustice are not uncommon (Baker and Smith 1991). Even though functional disability during the diagnostic phase is usually minimal, being diagnosed with PD is often viewed as a life-altering experience which can potentially threaten all aspects of life (Carter et al 1998).

The manner in which the diagnosis is conveyed is important, as this can potentially affect how the patient will respond (Phipps and Cuthill 2002). The diagnosis should be given in a sympathetic and understanding manner and the doctor should use language that the patient can easily understand. The patient should be given the opportunity to ask questions and should not be rushed. During this initial consultation the patient should be provided with as much or as little information about the disease course and its treatments as they desire.

Parkinson's disease Nurse Specialists (PDNSs) have a major role to play during the diagnostic phase of the disease as they can help facilitate acceptance of the diagnosis (Morgan and Moran 2001) through counselling and provision of appropriate and timely information (Noble 1998). Patients who do not receive information and education about their disease may display negative emotions towards their condition and towards healthcare professionals (Reid 2003). The main focus of nursing care at this stage in the disease should be to help patients accept the diagnosis and to empower them so that they are able to make informed decisions.

Accepting the diagnosis of PD can be particularly difficult for a younger person as the diagnosis may come when they are still developing their career, planning their financial security, raising a young family or even thinking about or starting a family (Parkinson's Disease Society 2002). In the UK, a useful resource for younger patients with PD is the special interest group YAPP&Rs (Young Alert Parkinson's, Partners & Relatives). Patients can contact YAPP&RS through the Parkinson's Disease Society (PDS) helpline or through their website (www.youngonset-parkinsons.org.uk). Similar groups are also available elsewhere.

Many PDNSs offer telephone support to patients and families and this can be especially valuable to newly diagnosed patients and their families, as they are sure to have many questions. Patient concerns vary considerably but common areas of concern include:

- Employment and financial issues
- Rate of progression
- Whether there is an hereditary basis to PD, i.e. will it affect my children?

- Effect on relationships, spouse and family
- Issues relating to driving

With the diagnosis of PD comes the role of the family caregiver (Carter et al 1998). Even though carer burden tends to be low in the early stages of the disease, some caregivers do experience a considerable amount of strain during this time (Carter et al 1998). It is not unusual for a spouse or partner to have difficulty accepting the diagnosis of PD and they may also experience feelings of anger, horror and denial. Additionally, they may have fears about the future and the potential impact the disease may have on their relationship with the patient. It is therefore important to inquire about the partner's concerns as well as the patient's.

Although disability is usually minimal during the diagnostic phase of the disease, some patients do experience functional difficulties such as slow hand function or slight difficulty in walking, and early referral to appropriate therapists can be beneficial.

Support groups such as the PDS can also be a great resource for newly diagnosed patients and families. Patients should be given their contact details and informed what support and resources that they can offer. The PDS offers a variety of resources including:

- Wide range of information sheets, booklets, audio tapes and videos on all aspects of PD
- Local support groups which offer mutual support, information, social activities and practical help at a local level
- Outreach service for black and minority ethnic communities
- Benefit advice
- Free phone helpline staffed by nurses

Support groups (not only for PD but also other movement disorders, including rarer forms of parkinsonism) offering similar services are available throughout the world. International listings and contact information of movement disorder support groups are available at www.wemove.org.

Summary

Although nurses usually have minimal contact with patients during the diagnostic phase of the disease it is important to have a basic understanding of the diagnostic workup, considerations and possible differential diagnoses. This helps the nurse to explain possible queries from patients and family members, as well as to be able to discuss alternative diagnoses with their physicians in cases where atypical features develop. Furthermore, nurses also have a huge role to play once the diagnosis has been confirmed in providing information about the disease and helping the patient to adjust to living with a chronic progressive illness.

Key points

- The main clinical features of PD include bradykinesia, rigidity, tremor and postural instability
- There are currently no biological markers available that will lead to a completely definite diagnosis of PD during life so PD is diagnosed entirely on clinical grounds
- It is important to be aware of symptoms and signs that may indicate atypical parkinsonism, since the latter often worsens prognosis and inadequate treatment may cause disabling adverse events
- The diagnosis of PD can have a major impact on patients, and emotions such as fear, isolation, guilt, anger and injustice are not uncommon
- The emphasis of nursing care during the diagnostic phase of the disease is to facilitate acceptance of the disease by providing access to counselling and information
- The PDS plays a key role in providing support, information and advice to newly diagnosed patients and their families

References

Albanese A, Bonuccelli U, Brefel C, Chaudhuri K R, Colosimo C, Eichhorn T, Melamed E, Pollak P, Van Laar T and Zappia M (2001) Consensus statement on the role of acute dopaminergic challenge in Parkinson's disease. Movement Disorders 16: 197–201.

Baker M and Smith P (1991) The social worker. In: F I Caird (ed.) Rehabilitation in Parkinson's Disease. London: Chapman & Hall.

Barker R, Duncan J and Lees A (1989) Subcutaneous apomorphine as a diagnostic test for dopaminergic responsiveness in parkinsonian syndromes. Lancet 1(8639): 675.

Bhatia K, Brooks D J and Burn D J (1998) Guidelines for the management of Parkinson's Disease. Hospital Medicine 59: 469–479.

Bonifati V, De Michele G, Lucking C B, Durr A, Fabrizio E, Ambrosio G, Vanacore N, De Mari M, Marconi R, Capus L, Breteler M M, Gasser T, Oostra B, Wood N, Agid Y, Filla A, Meco G and Brice A; Italian PD Genetics Study Group, French PD Genetics Study Group, European Consortium on Genetic Susceptibility in PD (2001) The parkin gene and its phenotype. Neurological Sciences 22: 51–52.

Bonnet A M, Loria Y, Sain-Hilaire M H, Lhermitte F, Agid Y (1987) Does long-term aggravation of Parkinson's disease result from nondopaminergic lesions? Neurology 37: 1539–1542.

Brooks D J (1998) The early diagnosis of Parkinson's Disease. Annals of Neurology 44:S10–18.

Brown R G, Jahanshahi M, Quinn N, Marsden C D (1990) Sexual function in patients with Parkinson's disease. Journal of Neurology, Neurosurgery and Psychiatry 53: 480–486.

Carr J (2002) Tremor in Parkinson's disease. Parkinsonism and Related Disorders 8: 223–234.

Carter J H, Stewart B J, Archbold P G, Inoue I, Jaglin J, Lannon M, Rost-Ruffner E, Tennis M, McDermott M P, Amyot D, Barter R, Cornelius L, Demong C, Dobson J, Duff J, Erickson J, Gardiner N, Gauger L, Gray P, Kanigan B, Kiryluk B, Lewis P, Mistura K, Malapira T, Pay M, Sheldon C, Winfield L, Wolfington-Shallow K, Zoog K and the Parkinson Study Group (1998) Living with a person who has Parkinson's disease: the spouse's perspective by stage of disease. Movement Disorders 13: 20–28.

Clarke C E and Davies P (2000) Systematic review of acute levodopa and apomorphine challenge tests in the diagnosis of idiopathic Parkinson's disease. Journal of Neurology, Neurosurgery and Psychiatry 69: 590–594.

Cummings J L (1992) Depression in Parkinson's disease: a review. American Journal of Psychiatry 149: 443–454.

Defer G L, Widner H, Marie R M, Remy P and Levivier M (1999) Core assessment program for surgical interventional therapies in Parkinson's disease (CAPSIT-PD). Movement Disorders 14: 572–584.

Deuschl G, Bain P and Brin M (1998) Consensus statement of the Movement Disorder Society on Tremor. Ad Hoc Scientific Committee. Movement Disorders 13 (Suppl 3): 2–23.

Dodel R, Höffken H, Möller J C, Bornschein B, Klockgether T, Behr T, Oertel W H and Siebert U (2003) Dopamine transporter imaging and SPECT in diagnostic workup of Parkinson's disease: a decision-analytic approach. Movement Disorders 18 (Suppl 7): S52–S62.

Doty R L, Deems D A and Stellar S (1988) Olfactory dysfunction in parkinsonism: a general deficit unrelated to neurologic signs, disease stage or disease duration. Neurology 38: 1237–1244.

Edwards L L, Quigley E M M and Pfeiffer R F (1992) Gastrointestinal dysfunction in Parkinson's disease: frequency and pathophysiology. Neurology 42: 726–732.

Errea J M, Ara J R, Aibar C and de Pedro-Cuesta J (1999) Prevalence of Parkinson's disease in lower Aragon, Spain. Movement Disorders 14: 596–604.

Esteguy M, Bonnet A M, Kefalos J, Lhermitte F and Agid Y (1985) Le test à la levodopa dans la maladie de Parkinson. Revue Neurologique (Paris) 141: 413–415.

Fahn S, Elton R L, members of the UPDRS Development Committee (1987) Unified Parkinson's Disease Rating Scale. In: S Fahn, C D Marsden, D B Calne and M Goldstein (eds.) Recent Developments in Parkinson's Disease, volume 2. Florham Park, New Jersey: Macmillan Healthcare Information pp. 153–163.

Fall P A, Axelson O, Fredriksson M, Hansson G, Lindvall B, Olsson J E, Granerus A K (1998) Age-standardized incidence and prevalence of Parkinson's disease in a Swedish community. Journal of Clinical Epidemiology 49: 637–641.

Ford B. Pain in Parkinson's disease. Clinical Neuroscience 5: 63–72.

Gasser T, Schwarz J, Arnold G, Trenkwalder C and Oertel W H (1992) Apomorphine test for dopaminergic responsiveness in patients with previously untreated Parkinson's disease. Archives of Neurology 49: 1131–1134.

Gelb D J, Oliver E and Gilman S (1999) Diagnostic criteria for Parkinson's disease. Archives of Neurology 56: 33–39.

Gibb W R G and Lees A J (1988) The relevance of the Lewy body to the pathogenesis of idiopathic Parkinson's disease. Journal of Neurology, Neurosurgery and Psychiatry 51: 745–752.

Gilman S (2002) Multiple system atrophy. In: J Jankovic, E Tolosa (eds.) Parkinson's Disease and Movement Disorders, 4th edition. Philadelphia: Lippincott Williams and Wilkins pp. 170–184.

Gilman S, Low P A, Quinn N, Albanese A, Ben-Shlomo Y, Fowler C J, Kaufmann H, Klockgether T, Lang A E, Lantos P L, Litvan I, Mathias C J, Oliver E, Robertson D, Schatz I and Wenning G K (1999) Consensus statement on the diagnosis of multiple system atrophy. Journal of Neurological Science 163: 94-98.

Glosser G (2001) Neurobehavioral aspects of movement disorders. Neurologic Clinics 19: 535–551.

Goldstein D S (2003) Dysautonomia in Parkinson's disease: neurocardiological abnormalities. Lancet Neurology 2: 669–676.

Hagell P (2000) Timed tests in clinical assessment of motor function in Parkinson's disease. Journal of Neuroscience Nursing 32: 331–336.

Hawkes C H, Shephard B C and Daniel S E (1997) Olfactory dysfunction in Parkinson's disease. Journal of Neurology, Neurosurgery and Psychiatry 62(5): 436–446.

Hoehn M M and Yahr M (1967) Parkinsonism: onset, progression and mortality. Neurology 5: 427–442.

Hornykiewicz O (1975) Parkinson's disease and its chemotherapy. Biochemical Pharmocology 24: 1061–1065.

Hubble J P (1997) Drug-induced parkinsonism. In: R L Watts, W C Koller (eds.) Movement Disorders: Neurologic Principles and Practice. New York: McGraw Hill, Inc, pp. 325–330.

Hughes A J (1999) Apomorphine test in the assessment of parkinsonian patients: a meta-analysis. Advances in Neurology 80: 363–368.

Hughes A J, Daniel S E, Kilford L and Lees A J (1992) Accuracy of clinical diagnosis of idiopathic Parkinson's disease: a clinicopathological study of 100 cases. Journal of Neurology, Neurosurgery and Psychiatry 55:181–184.

Hughes A J, Lees A J and Stern G M (1990) Apomorphine test to predict dopaminergic responsiveness in parkinsonian syndromes. Lancet 336: 32–34.

Hughes A J, Daniel S E and Lees A J (2001) Improved accuracy of clinical diagnosis of Lewy body Parkinson's disease. Neurology 57: 1497–1499.

Hughes A J, Daniel S E, Ben-Shlomo B and Lees A J (2002) The accuracy of diagnosis of parkinsonian syndromes in a specialist movement disorder service. Brain 125: 861–870.

Jankovic J (1992) Pathophysiology and clinical assessment of motor symptoms in Parkinson's disease. In: W C Koller (ed.) Handbook of Parkinson's Disease, 2nd edition. New York: Marcel Dekker Inc pp. 129–157.

Karlsen K, Larsen J P, Tandberg E and Jørgensen K (1999) Fatigue in patients with Parkinson's disease. Movement Disorders 14: 237–241.

Kumar R, Bergeron C and Lang A E (2002) Corticobasal degeneration. In: J Jankovic, E Tolosa (eds.) Parkinson's Disease and Movement Disorders, 4th edition. Philadelphia: Lippincott Williams and Wilkins pp. 185–198.

Kuopio A M, Marttila R J, Helenius H and Rinne U K (1999) Changing epidemiology of Parkinson's disease in southwestern Finland. Neurology 52: 302–308.

Lachenmayer L (2003) Differential diagnosis of parkinsonian syndromes: dynamics of time courses are essential. Journal of Neurology 250 (Suppl 1): 11–14.

Litvan I, Agid Y, Calne D, Campbell G, Dubois B, Duvoisin R C, Goetz C G, Golbe L I, Grafman J, Growdon J H, Hallett M, Jankovic J, Quinn N P, Tolosa E and Zee D S (1996) Clinical research criteria for the diagnosis of progressive supranuclear palsy (Steele-Richardson-Olszewski syndrome): report of the NINDS-SPSP international workshop. Neurology 47: 1–9.

Litvan I, Bhatia K P, Burn D J, Goetz C G, Lang A E, McKeith I, Quinn N, Sethi K D, Shults C, Wenning G K; Movement Disorders Society Scientific Issues Committee (2003) Movement Disorders Society Scientific Issues Committee report: SIC Task Force appraisal of clinical diagnostic criteria for parkinsonian disorders. Movement Disorders 18: 467–486.

Lyons K E, Pahwa R, Tröster A I and Koller W C (1997) A comparison of Parkinson's disease symptoms and self-reported functioning and well being. Parkinsonism and Related Disorders 3: 207–209.

Macphee G (2001) Diagnosis and differential diagnosis. In: J Playfer, J Hindle (eds.) Parkinson's Disease in the Older Patient. London: Arnold pp. 49–55.

Marsden C D (1994) Parkinson's disease. Journal of Neurology, Neurosurgery and Psychiatry 57: 672–681.

Marsden C D (1989) Slowness of movement in Parkinson's disease. Movement Disorders 4: 26–37.

McKeith I G, Galasko D, Kosaka K, Perry E K, Dickson D W, Hansen L A, Salmon D P, Lowe J, Mirra S S, Byrne E J, Lennox G, Quinn N P, Edwardson J A, Ince P G, Bergeron C, Burns A, Miller B L, Lovestone S, Collerton D, Jansen E N, Ballard C, de Vos R A, Wilcock G K, Jellinger K A and Perry R H (1996) Consensus guidelines for the clinical and pathologic diagnosis of dementia with Lewy bodies (DLB): report of the consortium on DLB international workshop. Neurology 47: 1113–1124.

McKeith I, Mintzer J, Aarsland D, Burn D, Chiu H, Cohen-Mansfield J, Dickson D, Dubois B, Duda J E, Feldman H, Gauthier S, Halliday G, Lawlor B, Lippa C, Lopez O L, Carlos Machado J, O'Brien J, Playfer J, Reid W; International Psychogeriatric Association Expert Meeting on DLB. Dementia with Lewy bodies. Lancet Neurology 3: 19–28.

Micieli G, Tosi P, Marcheselli S and Cavallini A. Autonomic dysfunction in Parkinson's disease. Neurological Sciences 24 (Suppl 1): S32–S34.

Morgan E and Moran M (2001) The Parkinson's disease nurse specialist. In: J R Playfer and J V Hindle (ed.) Parkinson's disease in the Older Patient. London: Arnold pp. 273–282.

Noble C (1998) Parkinson's Disease: the challenge. Nursing Standard 15(12): 43–51.

Pahwa R and Lyons K E (2003) Essential tremor: differential diagnosis and current therapy. American Journal of Medicine 115: 134–142.

Parkinson's Disease Society (2002) One in twenty: an information pack for younger people with parkinson's. Parkinson's Disease Society of the United Kingdom.

Phipps L L and Cuthill J D (2002) Breaking bad news: a clinician's view of the literature. Annals (Royal College of Physicians and Surgeons of Canada) 35(5): 287–293.

Poewe W and Scherfler C (2003) Role of dopamine transporter imaging in investigation of parkinsonian syndromes in clinical practice. Movement Disorders 18 (Suppl 7): S16–21.

Poewe W H and Wenning G K (1998) The natural history of Parkinson's disease. Annals of Neurology 44(Suppl 1): S1–9.

Pogarell O and Oertel W H (1999) Parkinsonian syndromes and Parkinson's disease. In: P Le Witt and W H Oertel (eds.) Parkinson's Disease: The Treatment Options. London: Martin Dunitz, pp. 1–10.

Quinn N P (1995) Parkinsonism: recognition and differential diagnosis. British Medical Journal 310: 447–452.

Quinn N P (1997) Parkinson's disease: clinical features. In: N P Quinn (ed.) Clinical Neurology: Parkinsonism. London: Baillière Tindall pp. 1–14.

Rajput A H, Rozdilsky B and Rajput A (1991) Accuracy of clinical diagnosis in parkinsonism: a prospective study. Canadian Journal of Neurological Science 18: 275–278.

Reid J (2003) Diagnosis of Parkinson's disease: why patient education matters. Professional Nurse 19(1): 33–35.

Riederer P and Wuketich S (1976) Time course of nigrostriatal degeneration in Parkinson's disease; a detailed study of influential factors in human brain analogues. Journal of Neural Transmission. Parkinson's Disease and Dementia Section 38: 277–301.

Riley D E and Lang A E (2000) Clinical diagnostic criteria. Advances in Neurology 82: 29–34.

Riley D, Lang A E, Blair R D, Birnbaum A and Reid B (1989) Frozen shoulder and other shoulder disturbances in Parkinson's disease. Journal of Neurology, Neurosurgery and Psychiatry 52: 63–66.

Rossi P, Colosimo C, Moro E, Tonali P and Albanese A (2000) Acute challenge with apomorphine and levodopa in Parkinsonism. European Neurology 43: 95–101.

Savoiardo M (2003) Differential diagnosis of Parkinson's disease and atypical parkinsonian disorders by magnetic resonance imaging. Neurological Sciences 24 (Suppl 1): S35–37.

Sawle G (1999) Parkinsonism: Parkinson's disease. In: G Sawle (ed.) Movement disorders in Clinical Practice. Oxford: Isis Medical Media Ltd pp. 7–33.

Schrag A, Ben-Shlomo Y and Quinn N P (2000) Cross sectional prevalence survey of idiopathic Parkinson's disease and parkinsonism in London. British Medical Journal 321: 21–22.

Schulman L M, Taback R L, Rabinstein A A and Weiner W J (2002) Non-recognition of depression and other non-motor symptoms in Parkinson's disease. Parkinsonism and Related Disorders 8: 193–197.

Swinn L, Schrag A, Viswanathan R, Bloem B R, Lees A and Quinn N (2003) Sweating dysfunction in Parkinson's disease. Movement Disorders 18: 1459–1463.

Taba P and Asser T (2002) Prevalence of Parkinson's disease in Estonia. Acta Neurologica Scandinavica 106: 276–281.

Taba P and Asser T (2003) Incidence of Parkinson's disease in Estonia. Neuroepidemiology 22: 41–45.

Tandberg E, Larsen J P, Nessler E G, Riise T and Aarli J A (1995) The epidemiology of Parkinson's disease in the county of Rogaland, Norway. Movement Disorders 10: 541–549.

Tolosa E, Valldeoriola F and Pastor P (2002) Progressive supranuclear palsy. In: J Jankovic, E Tolosa (eds.) Parkinson's Disease and Movement Disorders, 4th edition. Philadelphia: Lippincott Williams and Wilkins pp. 152–169.

van Hilten J J, Wagemans E A, Ghafoerkhan S F and van Laar T (1997) Movement characteristics in Parkinson's disease: determination of dopaminergic responsiveness and threshold. Clinical Neuropharmacology 20: 402–408.

Valls-Sole J (2000) Neurophysiological characterization of parkinsonian syndromes. Clinical Neurophysiology 30: 352–367.

Vines J J, Larumbe R, Gaminde I and Artazcoz M T (1999) Incidence of idiopathic and secondary Parkinson disease in Navarre. Population-based case registry. Neurologia 14: 16–22.

Vingerhoets F J G, Schulzer M, Calne D B and Snow B J (1997) Which clinical sign of Parkinson's disease best reflects the nigrostriatal lesion? Annals of Neurology 41: 58–64.

Wermuth L, Joensen P, Bunger N and Jeune B (1997) High prevalence of Parkinson's disease in the Faroe Islands. Neurology 49: 426–432.

Wermuth L, von Weitzel-Mudersbach P and Jeune B (2000) A two-fold difference in the age-adjusted prevalences of Parkinson's disease between the island of Als and the Faroe Islands. European Journal of Neurology 7: 655–660.

Winikates J and Jankovic J (1999) Clinical correlates of vascular parkinsonism. Archives of Neurology 56: 98–102.

Yamanouchi H and Nagura H (1997) Neurological signs and frontal white matter lesions in vascular parkinsonism. A clinicopathologic study. Stroke 28: 965–969.

Yekhlef F, Ballan G, Macia F, Delmer O, Sourgen C and Tison F (2003) Routine MRI for the differential diagnosis of Parkinson's disease, MSA, PSP, and CBD. Journal of Neural Transmission 110: 151–169.

CHAPTER THREE
Drug treatment of Parkinson's disease

JACQUI HANDLEY

Over the past 30 years tremendous progress has been made in the development of treatments for Parkinson's disease (PD), the main focus of which is drug therapy. Patients with PD experience a wide variety of symptoms and variable prognoses, so drug regimens have to be carefully and individually designed. There is also a need to balance benefit with side effects. In early disease this is relatively easy to achieve but as time progresses drugs may lose efficacy, symptoms become more intrusive and side effects become more common and troublesome. This detailed approach to drug regimens may be difficult for non-specialists to manage, but nurses, in particular nurse specialists, can be very effective in helping doctors to achieve optimum control. Patients and their carer or partner will also need to develop an understanding of their drug regimens in order to administer them accurately and to identify their treatment needs.

This chapter will discuss the different medications currently available to treat PD and it will also focus on nursing issues such as drug timing and administration, interaction with food, and patient understanding and compliance.

Introduction

When creating a treatment plan for a person with PD, drug therapy is described as the 'central pillar' (Playfer 2001) around which care is designed. A rational application of pharmaceutical principles will be required for determining a suitable regimen. However, the symptoms experienced and the response to drugs vary widely so drug regimens need to be custom made for the individual. LeWitt (1997) suggests that success depends on applying the art of medicine as much as the principles of science.

To date, all drugs used to treat PD are symptomatic in that they treat the symptoms but not the underlying cause. However, many new approaches are being developed and it is, therefore, reasonable to encourage patients to be optimistic about more proactive treatments being available in the future. The symptoms of PD occur as a result of depleted levels of the neurotransmitter dopamine (DA) and the central aim of treatment is to restore DA levels to as near normal as possible. However, at present there is no technology that allows exact determination of DA levels and deciding on the amount of treatment required depends on clinical judgement and experience.

Progression of the disease almost always brings disabling complications, some of which are directly attributable to the disease progression whilst others are the result of long-term treatments (Bhatia et al 1998). For this reason, it is often recommended that drug treatment should be withheld until the symptoms of the disease cause disability of practical significance to the individual (Olanow et al 2001). During the pre-drug phase, contact with a Parkinson's disease Nurse Specialist (PDNS), physiotherapist, occupational therapist, speech therapist and the Parkinson's Disease Society (PDS) can be helpful as they can provide support, information and health promotional advice. Many patients can be maintained without drugs for some time providing they have access to adequate support and information to help them understand the potential benefits of delaying drug therapy.

Burns (2002) recommends that any discussions about when to start treatment should consider factors such as the patient's age, severity of symptoms, cognitive impairment or other neuropsychiatric features, as well as social factors, such as threatened loss of employment, loss of ability to drive, therapeutic cost and the expectations of the individual and their family. An assessment of other factors, such as the likelihood of falls and whether there is existing concurrent illness, should also be considered. Once the decision to start drug treatment has been made, most doctors will follow either local or national guidelines (Bhatia et al 2001). Burns (2002) suggests that although recent national guidelines provide an excellent review of the strategies available there is still a lack of researched evidence to recommend one drug over another. The specific needs of the individual must therefore be the most important guiding factor.

Drugs in current use

Currently 18 drugs are licensed in the UK for the treatment of PD (BNF 2002). These can be categorized into four main groups (PDS 1999):

- Drugs that replace DA – levodopa
- Drugs that prevent the breakdown of DA – catechol-*O*-methyltransferase (COMT) and monoamine oxidase type B (MAOB) inhibitors
- Drugs that mimic the action of levodopa – DA agonists
- Drugs that block the action of acetylcholine – anticholinergics

Levodopa

Dopamine itself cannot be administered to replenish depleted striatal DA levels as it is not orally active, is rapidly broken down and is unable to cross the blood–brain barrier (BBB). However, levodopa is the precursor to DA and this amino acid is orally active and able to cross the BBB. Once levodopa has entered the brain it is converted to DA by the enzyme dopa-decarboxylase. Levodopa has been the mainstay of drug treatment for PD for over 30 years and has been referred to as the gold standard treatment (Playfer 2001). Levodopa gives the best ratio of benefit versus side effects of all the anti-Parkinson's drugs (Oertel and Quinn 1997). A list of the different levodopa preparations currently available in the UK is shown in Table 3.1. It is not unusual for patients to take a combination of standard, dispersible and controlled-release preparations in an attempt to control their symptoms.

In the early stages of PD most people benefit from levodopa treatment. It is especially helpful in improving bradykinesia and rigidity but is less so in treating tremor (Playfer 2001). Abrupt withdrawal of levodopa is not recommended as this can induce a rare life-threatening condition known as malignant levodopa withdrawal syndrome.

Table 3.1 Levodopa preparations available

Co-beneldopa (Madopar)	
Standard release	*Controlled release*
62.5 mg capsule	125 mg capsule
125 mg capsule	250 mg capsule
62.5 mg dispersible tablet	
125 mg dispersible tablet	
Co-careldopa (Sinemet)	
Standard release	*Controlled release*
62.5 mg tablet	Half-CR (125 mg) tablet
110 mg tablet	CR (250 mg) tablet
Plus (125 mg) tablet	
Sinemet 275	

Until recently, a trial of levodopa was often used as a diagnostic tool (see pp. 18–19). Although this practice is no longer recommended, Quinn (1995) suggests that when a patient does not show a good initial response to levodopa the diagnosis should be questioned.

Limitations of levadopa

Although levodopa remains the main treatment for PD, some serious limitations have emerged including its short mode of action, neuropsychiatric complications and the emergence of dyskinesias (involuntary movements).

Short mode of action

The short mode of action of levodopa relates to its short half-life and to the gradually diminishing ability of the presynaptic nerve terminals to store DA as the disease progresses (Playfer 2001). This results in end-of-dose deterioration and 'wearing off'. The terms 'on' and 'off' are frequently used in managing PD. LeWitt (1997) describes an 'on' state as when the drugs are working and an 'off' state as when they are not. Perceptions of an 'on' state and an 'off' state vary widely. In the early stages of treatment the motor state will usually vary gently, but over time an 'all or nothing' response to a dose of levodopa is likely to develop. Once the patient develops motor fluctuations the process cannot usually be reversed; much of the focus of modern PD treatment is on this issue. Motor fluctuations are discussed in more depth in Chapter 4.

Neuropsychiatric problems

Neuropsychiatric problems may occur with levodopa, particularly in elderly people and those with complex forms of PD, such as Lewy body disease. Neuropsychiatric complications can include sleep disturbance, vivid dreams, hallucinations, delusions or organic confusional psychosis (Hindle 2001). Minimizing these complications may require an overall reduction in PD medications but Hindle (2001) suggests that, since levodopa is probably the least hallucinogenic of all the PD drugs and perhaps the most effective, it should be the last to be reduced.

Dyskinesias

Dyskinesias are likely to occur within 3–5 years of starting treatment (Playfer 2001). At present, there are few drugs available to treat dyskinesias and the most effective way to resolve them is to reduce the dosage of levodopa. However, this may result in an unacceptable re-emergence of the PD symptoms. To manage these it is recommended that levodopa should be used at lower doses than in the past (Olanow et al 2001).

Catechol-*O*-methyltransferase (COMT) inhibitors

COMT is an enzyme that is systemically distributed and normally converts much of the ingested levodopa dose to a non-toxic metabolite called 3-*O*-methyldopa. Inhibition of this enzyme allows the achievement of more stable and sustained plasma levodopa levels, which increases the amount of levodopa that enters the brain (Rinne et al 1998). This may allow lower doses of levodopa to be used without any loss of treatment benefit.

There is one COMT inhibitor currently available in the UK: entacapone (Comtess). This is a peripheral COMT inhibitor and it must be administered along with a dose of levodopa. Hubble (2002) suggests that a major advantage of this drug is that it can be introduced relatively easily without the need for gradual dose escalation.

The side effects most commonly experienced with entacapone, dyskinesias and nausea, are similar to those of levodopa as they relate to increased dopaminergic (DA-ergic) activity. These can usually be managed by reducing the daily levodopa dose, perhaps by 15–30% (Olanow et al 2001). Patients should be informed that entacapone might discolour their urine or cause mild diarrhoea.

Monoamine oxidase type B (MAOB) inhibitors

Selegiline is an MAOB inhibitor which readily crosses the BBB. Inhibition of MAOB results in a slower breakdown of DA and thus prolongs the central activity of DA (Swale 1999). Selegiline has a long half-life and produces metabolites which can cause insomnia, hallucinations and vivid dreams. Whilst selegiline is well tolerated as monotherapy, when used in conjunction with other DA-ergic drugs it can increase dyskinesias and neuropsychiatric complications (Olanow and Obeso 2000).

Zelapar is a newer formulation of selegiline which is absorbed sublingually. This method of administration allows a reduced dose to be administered compared with the dose of standard selegiline and thus it is associated with fewer side effects. Zelapar is particularly useful for those with swallowing difficulties and those who suffer side effects with standard selegiline.

For many years selegiline was used in early disease and was thought to have neuroprotective properties (Olanow et al 1998). This is now considered unlikely but the debate continues and selegiline remains in general use.

Dopamine agonists

Waters (1999) describes DA agonists as 'the most effective drugs for treating Parkinson's with the exception of levodopa'. DA agonists act on pre- and postsynaptic DA receptors. There are two main types of DA receptors, D1-like (D1 and D5) and D2-like (D2, D3 and D4), and DA agonists tend to be specific for certain receptors. There are six oral agonists currently licensed for use in the UK (Table 3.2). Apomorphine is an additional DA agonist which can only be administered by subcutaneous injection and this drug is covered separately in Chapter 5.

Table 3.2 Dopamine agonists currently available in the UK

Bromocriptine (Parlodel)	Ergot. Acts on D2 receptors. Half-life 2–6 hours
Lisuride	Ergot. Acts on D1 and D2 receptors. Short acting
Pergolide (Celance)	Ergot. Acts on D1 and D2 receptors. Half-life 4–6 hours
Cabergoline (Cabaser)	Ergot. Acts on D2 receptors. Once daily dose as long half-life (63–68 hours)
Ropinirole (Requip)	Non-ergot. Acts on D2 and D3 receptors
Pramipexole (Mirapexin)	Non-ergot. Acts on D2 and D3 receptors. Half-life 12 hours

There are several theoretical advantages for using DA agonists which include:

- Direct action, which is independent of the degenerating neurons
- More reliable absorption and transport to the brain than levodopa
- Longer half-life than levodopa
- No generation of free radicals or induction of oxidative stress
- Possible neuroprotective qualities, which may slow down disease progression (Schapira 2002)

Although the last factor is extremely exciting in terms of long-term outcomes for patients, there are some difficulties in using DA agonists in practice, particularly with elderly patients. Older people have a slower metabolism and the half-life, or the time taken for plasma levels to reduce by half following complete absorption of the drug, can be extended (Strachan 2001). The longer half-life of DA agonists can lead to drug accumulation causing high plasma concentrations which may result in toxicity and side effects. The main side effects of all of the agonists are:

- Neuropsychiatric complications, in particular hallucinations and impaired cognition
- Sleep disturbance and excessive daytime somnolence
- Postural hypotension

Whilst all the agonists have a similar mode of action they emerge as slightly different when used in practice and if one proves intolerable or ineffective other agonists should be tried (Playfer 2001).

In recent years concerns have been raised about PD patients who drive, as sudden-onset daytime somnolence or 'sleep episodes' have been reported in a number of patients taking DA agonists (Frucht et al 1999). This raised questions about whether patients taking DA agonists should be allowed to drive, but it has now been recognized that all of the DA-ergic drugs, including levodopa, can have this effect (Pirker and Happe 2000). All patients with PD who drive should be informed of the risk of sudden onset somnolence and informed that they should not drive if they experience this side effect. Patients in the titration period, taking high doses of agonists, on additional sedative drugs and of advanced age or disease duration (Pal et al 2001) need to be particularly cautious.

Anticholinergics

Anticholinergic drugs were first used to treat PD by Charcot in the 19th century in the form of belladonna. Anticholinergics block interstriatal cholinergic transmission. This helps to restore the balance of activity between the cholinergic and DA-ergic systems which become imbalanced as a result of the DA loss. The anticholinergic drugs currently available in the UK are:

- Benzhexol hydrochloride
- Benztropine mesylate
- Biperiden
- Orphenadrine hydrochloride
- Procyclidine hydrochloride

Anticholinergics are especially effective at treating tremor but tolerance can be a major issue as many patients experience neuropsychiatric side effects when taking these drugs (Sarter and Bruno 1998). Olanow and others (2001) recommend that anticholinergics should be used only occasionally and only as early therapy for young patients with tremor-dominant disease. In addition to the neuropsychiatric side effects, peripheral parasympathomimetic side effects such as glaucoma, dry mouth, blurred vision, urinary retention and constipation may occur (Bhatia et al 1998).

Amantadine

Amantadine could be described as belonging to a separate group of drugs as its mode of action is largely unknown. However, it is known that amantadine can increase DA release and inhibit DA uptake (Bhatia et al 1998). Amantadine has been used as an early PD treatment for around 30 years and it has recently been demonstrated as an effective treatment for dyskinesias (Verhagen et al 1998). The last daily dose of amantadine should be taken before 4pm in order to avoid sleep disturbance. If it is used to treat dyskinesias in later disease, higher doses of up to 600 mg may be required (Lees 2001). Withdrawal of amantadine should be gradual to avoid weight loss, cognitive impairment, hallucinations, fluid retention and vasculitis (Uitti et al 1996).

Nursing issues

Although nurses do not, to date, prescribe drugs for treating PD, many will be involved in drug administration, either in hospital or in the community. Some issues take on particular significance, such as timing of doses, patient understanding and compliance, interactions with food and changing the drug regimen.

Timing of drug administration

As the response to drugs is so variable, a truly individual regimen needs to be devised for each patient. In order that this regimen achieves optimum balance between benefit and side effects, the patient, and perhaps the partner or carer, must be an active participant in discussions about what to use and when. Timing can be particularly significant for achievement of steady plasma DA levels as this is required for optimum relief of symptoms.

In late-stage PD, particularly when long-acting drugs cannot be tolerated, achieving optimum control may necessitate frequent dosing with levodopa, perhaps every 1–2 hours. Frequent dosing may be necessary to gain symptom relief, but it can be difficult to achieve when the patient is admitted into hospital or for respite care. When the patient is away from home normal drug regimens are essential to maintain good control and engender patient confidence. However, errors and delays can occur and this can result in a very anxious and perhaps immobile patient. This problem is highlighted so frequently by patients that the PDS have raised it as a recent point for national action. One idea is for hospital nurses to use timers as reminders to administer tablets. Self-administration schemes can be effective but may be unsuitable when the patient is very unwell, is cognitively impaired or has been admitted for complex medication changes. When planning discharge, consideration must be given to how patients will administer complex regimens at home. Pre-prepared drug administrations systems such as Nomad or Dossett boxes can be helpful.

While frequent dosing can be difficult for others to maintain it is suggested that allowing patients to control the exact timing of their medication can be therapeutic, giving them a feeling of control (Hurtig

1994). This is particularly true in early disease as people try to come to terms with their diagnosis and the possibilities of increasing disability. Many doctors therefore encourage a degree of flexibility in drug regimens, over timing of doses and the opportunity to include an occasional extra 'rescue' dose. Although this works with most patients it can lead to the development of a disorder known as hedonistic homeostatic dysregulation (Giovannoni et al 2000), or dopamine-addictive behaviours similar to those associated with substance misuse and addiction. To avoid these problems drug regimens should be designed with carefully defined boundaries and a maximum daily dose (Hurtig 1994). Although the severe states are uncommon, many patients and carers describe their lives as 'governed by pills' with their complex regimens and frequent doses.

Patient understanding and compliance

In order for patients to contribute to decisions about their drug regimens they need to understand the symptoms of PD and the treatment options available. PDNSs were first introduced in 1988 and education of patients and carers has become one of the core duties of the role (MacMahon 1998). With education and information presented in appropriate language, in interesting formats and at the appropriate time, patients can be assisted to become 'expert' in managing their disease. Such expertise has been shown to lead to better control of symptoms as a result of improved drug compliance and to help the psychological processes which lead to an acceptance of having PD (Harris et al 1998).

Compliance with drug regimens is very important because some of the drugs are very short-acting and combination therapy is often required. Poor understanding of drug side effects and disease symptoms can lead to poor compliance and poor decision-making about whether to increase or decrease tablets. Koller (1999) suggests that there is also a particular need to learn the difference between tremor and dyskinesias. Patients must be taught to recognize symptoms and side effects, and this information may need to be reiterated on many occasions, as symptoms and side effects change as the disease progresses. Koller (1999) also stresses the importance of education and support for the patient's partner, as a misinformed, unhappy partner can have such an adverse effect on drug compliance that the overall management of PD can deteriorate.

With each new drug added to the regimen the risk of side effects increases, as does the risk of poor compliance. A study of 170 patients with PD found that when three different drugs were used 20% of the doses were taken incorrectly; when 10 different drugs were used almost 100% were taken incorrectly (Reid and Stewart 2000). As 26.5% of the study population had at least five medications prescribed, the conclusions were that people being treated for PD were at significant risk of poor compliance. Multi-dosing, combination therapy and co-morbid conditions were also found to have an adverse effect on compliance. As all of these issues are common in PD, along with cognitive decline, it must be acknowledged that drug compliance is a major concern in daily practice.

Interactions with food

Patients often ask whether they should take their PD medication with or without food. When drugs are first introduced pharmacists' and manufacturers' information sheets advise taking doses after meals as a strategy to combat the common early side effects of nausea and vomiting. All DA-ergic drugs can cause nausea as they activate the vomiting centre through medullary neurons in the chemoreceptor trigger zone. Most people quickly develop tolerance to drug-induced nausea and should be advised to take small meals or snacks with each dose. Some patients need treatment with an antiemetic, such as domperidone, until tolerance has developed. Domperidone is a peripheral D2 receptor antagonist and is the only antiemetic recommended for people with PD. Other antiemetics, such as metoclopramide and prochlorperazine, can block both central and peripheral DA receptors and therefore increase PD symptoms. Domperidone should not be used long term but it can be reintroduced to susceptible patients when introducing new drugs.

Many patients who have taken levodopa for some time report that their dose of co-beneldopa or co-careldopa is less effective when taken after a large or high-protein meal. This is because large neutral amino acids have to compete with levodopa for active transport from the duodenum into the blood stream, leading to reduced levodopa plasma levels and decreased cerebral availability (Swale 1999). For these patients it is recommended that levodopa be taken 30–40 minutes before mealtimes (Playfer 2001) or 1–2 hours afterwards. However, in some patients this may induce dyskinesias that are sufficiently disabling to make eating difficult, and further experimentation with timing may be required (Frankel et al 1989). In contrast to the effect that food can have on standard-release levodopa, it has been suggested that if controlled-release preparations are taken with food the bioavailability is increased and therefore the action will be enhanced (Djaldetti et al 1996). A new form of levodopa, levodopa ethylester, is currently being tested in clinical trials (Djaldetti et al 2002). This is available as an oral solution, which is highly soluble and might overcome the impaired absorption problems of current levodopa preparations.

DA agonists are not subject to competition with food for absorption and can therefore be taken with meals without loss of action. However, there is some evidence that when taken with food their action may be delayed for up to 4 hours (Thalamas et al 1996). The quest to achieve control throughout the day can be very critical, particularly for those with advanced disease, and an exact history of timings of drug doses and meals should be taken. The process of building this picture can be helped significantly if the patient can complete a diary that includes 'on/off' states and meal and drug times over a period of several days.

As well as problems with absorption of drugs, some people with advanced PD experience problems with gastric emptying which may lead to an unpredictable response to medication and fluctuations in control.

Making changes

As drug treatments for PD are currently only aimed at treating symptoms, the disease process remains unaffected and the patient will, in time, require more treatment to control the symptoms. Services for people with PD must therefore include regular reviews in order to monitor changes and adjust treatments to achieve optimum symptom control. Patients can be taught to recognize when change is necessary but they will always need to acknowledge the necessary compromise between short- and long-term needs and the risk:benefit ratio of therapies (Koller 1999).

The clinical consequences of any change in levodopa therapy can take 2 weeks to become apparent, and with DA agonists it may take months to establish a regimen (Olanow et al 2001). Changes to PD regimens should be made in the outpatient setting whenever possible, as hospital inpatient facilities can rarely provide this timescale (LeWitt 1997).

PDNSs can be particularly effective at monitoring drug changes as most are able to work across primary and secondary care and can act as a link between consultant outpatient clinics, GPs and the patient at home. At present, PDNSs are not able to prescribe drugs but their role includes assessment of the individual's needs and liaison with medical staff on the most appropriate treatment strategy. If possible simple, perhaps non-drug related, changes should be made first, but when major change is required this must be made in accordance with agreed local policy. It should always be remembered that the person who signs the prescription retains legal responsibility for their actions in providing that medication (Holmes 2001). Although PDNSs are not responsible for the initial prescription, some are able to make slight changes by following local policy on titration of new drugs and changing existing regimens. As the role of PDNSs challenges established boundaries between the medical and the nursing roles, they should pay particular attention to ensure their practice conforms to local policy. However, it is recognized that conforming with current legislation may prove unwieldy in practice; it is widely acknowledged that change in legislation on nurse prescribing is long overdue (DOH 1999).

When discussing changes in drug regimens it is impossible to list all the possible actions that could be tried in view of the myriad of individual needs and the number of drugs available. The following points are a few basic principles which should be applied regardless of the change made, by whom or when.

- Changes to a regimen should only be made following a detailed discussion with the patient and, perhaps, carer
- A careful assessment of physical and psychosocial needs should be made: change is not always appropriate
- Treatment guidelines should be followed, where possible, but individual circumstances must be taken into account
- Changes, either to stop or introduce new tablets, should be made gradually in order to develop tolerance, minimize side effects and optimize control
- The importance of the drug regimen and the significance of any change to the patient must be recognized. Many patients feel more vulnerable when change is necessary and need extra support and reassurance at this time
- Nurses, in particular PDNSs, must be clear on prescribing legislation and act according to agreed local policy

Key points

- All drugs used to treat PD treat the symptoms and not the underlying cause of the disease
- Drugs for PD can be categorized into four groups: levodopa, COMT and MAOB inhibitors, DA agonists and anticholinergics
- Nurses have an important role to play in educating patients about their medications and informing them about important factors such as taking their medication on time and interactions with food

References

Bhatia K, Brooks D and Burn D J (1998) Guidelines for the management of Parkinson's disease. Hospital Medicine 59(6): 469–480.

Bhatia K, Brooks D, Burn D J, Clarke C E, Grossett D, MacMahon D, Playfer J, Schapira A, Stewart D and Williams A (2001) Updated guidelines for the management of Parkinson's disease. Hospital Medicine 62: 456–470.

British National Formulary (2002) Drugs used in Parkinsonism and related disorders. BNF March 43 Section 4.9. London: BMA pp. 239–246.

Burns D (2002) Treatment guidelines for Parkinson's disease: what's new? Prescriber 6(1): 20–23.

Carlsson A (2002) Role of dopamine in psychiatric and neurological disorders. Progress in Neurology and Psychiatry 6(3): 11–20.

Department of Health (1999) Review of Prescribing, Supply and Administration of Medicines: Final Report (Crown). London: DOH.

Djaldetti R, Baron J, Ziv I and Melamed E (1996) Gastric emptying in Parkinson's disease: Patients with and without response fluctuations. Neurology 46: 1051–1054.

Djaldetti R, Inzelberg R, Giladi N, Korczyn A D, Peretz-Aharon Y, Rabey M J, Herishano Y, Homigman S, Badarny S and Melamed E (2002) Oral solution of levadopa ethylester for treatment of response fluctuations in patients with advanced Parkinson's disease. Movement Disorders 17(2): 297–302.

Ferreira J, Galitzky M, Montastruc J L and Rascol O (2000) Sleep attacks in Parkinson's disease. Lancet 355: 1333–1334.

Frankel J P, Kempster P A, Bovingdon M, Webster R, Lees A J and Stern G M (1989) The effects of oral protein on the absorption of intraduodenal L-dopa and performance. Journal of Neurology, Neurosurgery and Psychiatry 52: 1063–1067.

Frucht S, Rogers M D, Greene P E, Gordon M F and Fahn S (1999) Falling asleep at the wheel: motor vehicle mishaps in persons taking pramipexole and ropinirole. Neurology 52: 1908–1910.

Giovannoni G, O'Sullivan J D and Turner K (2000) Hedonistic homeostatic dysregulation in patients with Parkinson's disease on dopamine replacement therapies. Journal of Neurology, Neurosurgery and Psychiatry 68(4): 423–428.

Harris K, Osbourne L, Richards K and Stewart J (1998) Education for patients with Parkinson's disease. British Journal of Community Nursing 3(5): 221–225.

Hindle J V (2001) Neuropsychiatry. In: J Playfer and J Hindle (eds.) Parkinson's Disease in the Older Patient. London: Arnold pp. 106–133.

Holmes S (2001) An introduction to GP prescribing and the law. Prescriber 19.2.01: 43–49.

Hubble J P (2002) Long-term studies of dopamine agonists. Neurology 58 (4 suppl 1): S33–41.

Hurtig H (1994) The doctor–patient relationship in chronic illness. In: M Stern (ed.) Beyond the Decade of the Brain. Tunbridge Wells: Wells Medical, pp. 73–88.

Koller W C (1999) Drug treatment for Parkinson's disease: impact on the patient's quality of life. In: P Martin and W Koller (eds.) Quality of Life in Parkinson's Disease. Barcelona: Masson pp. 79–92.

Koller W C (2002) Treatment of early Parkinson's disease. Neurology 58 (suppl 1): S79–86.

Lees A (2001) New advances in the management of late stage Parkinson's disease. Advances in Clinical Neuroscience and Rehabilitation 1(4): 7–8.

LeWitt P (1997) New options for treatment of Parkinson's disease. In: N Quinn (ed.) Parkinsonism. London: Baillière-Tindall pp. 109–123.

MacMahon D (1998) Practical approach to quality of life in Parkinson's disease: the nurse's role. Journal of Neurology 245(suppl 1): 19–22.

Metman L V, Del Dotto P, LePoole K, Konitsiotis S, Fang J and Chase T N (1998) Amantadine as a treatment for dyskinesia and motor fluctuations in Parkinson's disease. Neurology 50: 1323–1326.

Nutt J G and Holford N H G (1996) Response to levadopa in Parkinson's disease: imposing pharmacological law and order. Annals of Neurology 39: 561–573.

Oertel W and Quinn N (1997) Parkinson's disease: drug therapy. In: N Quinn (ed.) Parkinsonism. London: Baillière-Tindall pp. 89–108.

Olanow C W, Myllyla V V and Sotaniemi K A (1998) Current status of selegiline as a neuro–protective agent in Parkinson's disease. Movement Disorders 13 (suppl 3): 55–58.

Olanow C W and Obeso J A (2000) Pulsatile stimulation of dopamine receptors and levadopa induced complications in Parkinson's disease: implications for early use of COMT inhibitors. Neurology 55 (suppl 4): S72–77.

Olanow C W, Watts R L and Koller W C (2001) An algorithm (decision tree) for the management of Parkinson's disease: treatment and guidelines. Neurology 56 (suppl 5): S1–88.

Pal S, Bhattacharya K F, Agapito C and Ray Chaudhuri K (2001) A study of excessive daytime sleepiness and its clinical significance in three groups of Parkinson's disease patients taking Pramipexole, Cabergoline and levadopa monotherapy. Journal of Neural Transmission 108(1): 71–77.

Parkinson's Disease Society (1999) Drug Management. PDS Nurse Pack Section 3 11–14.

Pahwa R, Lyons K and McGuire D (1996) Early morning akinesia in Parkinson's disease: effects of standard carbidopa/levadopa and sustained release. Neurology 46: 1059–1062.

Playfer J (2001) Drug therapy in Parkinson's disease. In: J Playfer and J Hindle (eds.) Parkinson's Disease in the Older Patient. London: Arnold pp. 283–308.

Pirker W and Happe S (2000) Sleep attacks in Parkinson's disease. Lancet 356: 597–600.

Quinn N (1995) Parkinson's disease – recognition and differential diagnosis. British Medical Journal 310: 447–452.

Rascol O and Ferreira J (2000) Prevention and therapeutic strategies for levadopa–induced dyskinesia in Parkinson's disease. Current Opinion in Neurology 13(4): 431–436.

Reid D and Stewart D (2000) Polypharmacy in Parkinson's disease. Progress in Neurology and Psychiatry 15: 15–16.

Rinne U K, Larsen J P, Siden A and Worm-Peterson J (1998) Entacapone enhances the response to levodopa in parkinsonian patients with motor fluctuations. Neurology 51(5): 1309–1314.

Sarter M and Bruno J P (1998) Corticol acetylcholine, reality distortion, schizophrenia and Lewy body dementia: too much or too little cortical acetylcholine? Brain Cognition 38: 297–316.

Schapira A H (2002) Neuroprotection and dopamine agonists. Neurology 58(4 suppl 1): S33–41.

Strachan S (2001) Medicines and older people: a nurse's guide to administration. British Journal of Community Nursing 6(6): 297–301.

Swale G (1999) Movement Disorders in Clinical Practice. Oxford: Isis Medical Media.

Thalamas C, Rayet C and Brefel C (1996) Effects of food on the pharmokinetics of ropinirole in patients with Parkinson's disease. Movement Disorders 11 (suppl 1): 138.

Uitti R J, Rajput A H and Ahlskog J E (1996) Amantadine treatment is an independent predictor of improved survival in Parkinson's disease. Neurology 46: 1551–1556.

Verhagen Metman L, Del Dotto P, van den Munckhof P, Fang J, Mouradian M M and Chase T N (1998) Amantadine as a treatment for dyskinesia and motor fluctuation in Parkinson's disease. Neurology 50: 1323–1326.

Waters C H (1999) Diagnosis and Management of Parkinson's Disease. Columbia: Professional Communications.

CHAPTER FOUR
Motor fluctuations

LESLEY SWINN

Introduction

Parkinson's disease (PD) is a variable and individual disease, but sooner or later most patients will develop motor fluctuations in response to their medication. Motor fluctuations are a complication of drug treatment and it is estimated that 40% of patients will develop them within 4–6 years of taking levodopa (Ahlskog and Muenter 2001). The emergence of motor fluctuations marks a crucial point in the disease, as it is often at this stage that patients will start to report increased difficulties with daily living, increased disability and increased dependence on others. The management of motor fluctuations is not easy and they present a difficult challenge to even the most experienced of PD specialists.

Motor fluctuations manifest themselves in a variety of ways and this chapter will discuss the following in turn:

- End of dose wearing-off
- 'On/off' fluctuations
- Dyskinesias
- Dystonia
- Freezing
- Unpredictable 'on/off' fluctuations
- Non-motor 'off' period symptoms

The chapter will also discuss issues such as the importance of patient and family participation and education, the assessment of motor fluctuations and the role of the nurse.

When to start levodopa?

The stage in the disease when the patient should start levodopa remains controversial (Factor 2001; Katzenschlager and Lees 2002); increasingly,

PD specialists are recommending therapeutic strategies designed to delay the onset of levodopa treatment and thus delay the onset of levodopa-related motor complications (Jankovic 2002). Most patients will eventually need to take levodopa as other therapeutic approaches will not provide them with adequate motor control. It is important that patients are given balanced, clear information about the various therapeutic options available so that they are able to make an informed decision which is based on facts and considers their individual circumstances and expectations.

Honeymoon effect

During the first few years of starting levodopa most patients experience a constant improvement in their motor symptoms despite only taking levodopa two or three times a day. This is often referred to as the 'honeymoon' period.

In early disease, the surviving dopaminergic (DA-ergic) neurones within the brain are still able to store dopamine (DA) (taken orally as levodopa then converted to DA in the brain) and release it under normal control. This usually results in a constant improvement in the patient's motor symptoms as there is a continuous supply of DA available to postsynaptic DA receptors. Unfortunately, as the disease progresses the brain loses the ability to store DA, owing to progressive loss of DA-ergic neurons. Consequently the postsynaptic DA receptors are exposed to swings in the levels of DA and motor fluctuations emerge.

End of dose wearing-off

The wearing-off effect is often the first motor fluctuation to emerge. Usually the first sign of wearing-off is that patients will notice that the effect of the bedtime levodopa dose has worn off when they wake up in the morning and consequently they experience morning stiffness and slowness. Gradually patients will start to experience wearing-off symptoms with daytime doses as well.

Wearing-off symptoms occur when plasma levodopa levels, and consequently brain DA levels, are low. There is a wide range of treatment options available to treat wearing-off and these include increasing the frequency of levodopa dosing, using long-acting levodopa preparations and addition of a DA agonist or a catechol-*O*-methyltranferase (Alder 2002).

'On/off' fluctuations

After several years of taking levodopa many patients will start to experience more sudden fluctuations in their motor response to levodopa; this is usually referred to as the 'on/off' phenomenon. The change from being mobile to immobile has been compared with the operation of an internal switch, hence the term 'on/off'.

The term 'on' refers to periods of good motor control and reflects optimal levels of plasma levodopa and DA stimulation within the brain. The term 'off' refers to periods of poor motor control and occurs when the plasma levodopa level and brain DA stimulation within the brain are subtherapeutic. Figure 4.1 illustrates the relationship between plasma levodopa levels and 'on/off' states.

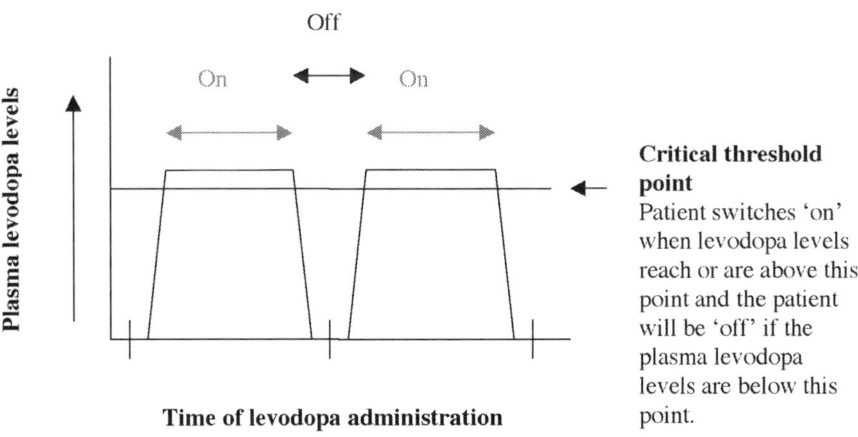

Figure 4.1 Relationship between 'on' and 'off' states and plasma levodopa levels.

It is very important to bear in mind that each patient's functional ability in the 'on' and the 'off' state can vary considerably. The transition time from the 'on' phase to the 'off' phase can also vary greatly. Most patients will experience a gradual worsening of their symptoms before they switch 'off', but some may switch between the 'on' and the 'off' state within a few seconds. Patients with advanced disease are more likely to experience rapid fluctuations and these can be extremely troublesome for both patients and carers. Those who experience rapid motor fluctuations should be advised to carry their medication with them at all times as this will ensure that they always have the ability to switch themselves back 'on'. Patients who live alone might benefit from having an alarm link system installed in their home to enable them to summon help if they switch 'off' and are unable to access their medication.

Most patients are usually able to predict when they are going to switch 'on' and 'off', especially in the earlier stages of the disease, as they know approximately how long each dose of levodopa will last. Many patients plan their daily activities around the times they are 'on'. The timing of administration and dosage of levodopa are important factors which determine when the patient is going to switch 'on' and 'off'. Most would like to be 'on' 100% of the time and for some this is achievable, especially in the early stages of the disease. However, as the disease advances, the balance between providing optimal motor control and minimizing side effects becomes more difficult and many patients may have to accept being 'off' for some of the time. The 'off' state can be unpleasant as it is often associated with pain, anxiety and loss of independence.

Patients should be encouraged to take their medication at prescribed times, as delayed administration may result in unnecessary 'off' time. Some patients, especially those with frequent dosing, develop strategies to ensure that they take their medication on time. 'Clock watching', the use of pill timers or merely relying on their carers to remind them when their medication is due are frequently employed strategies. There are a variety of pill timers available which can be purchased from most chemists.

Dyskinesias

The term dyskinesias refers to involuntary writhing movements. Dyskinesias are a common complication of levodopa therapy and typically occur when levodopa levels in the blood and brain are at their peak (peak-dose dyskinesias). However, patients can also experience dyskinesias when their plasma levodopa is at an intermediate level and these are referred to as biphasic dyskinesias. Biphasic dyskinesias generally occur when the levodopa levels are falling or rising, either at the beginning of the levodopa cycle or at the end. Biphasic dyskinesias predominantly affect younger patients and tend to be more violent in nature than peak-dose dyskinesias. Figure 4.2 illustrates the relationship between levodopa levels and peak-dose and biphasic dyskinesias.

Dyskinesias are common but there appears to be no general consensus as to their prevalence (Ahlskog and Meunter 2001). However, it is generally accepted that about 10% of patients on levodopa develop dyskinesias each year; Olanow and Koller (1998) estimated that 50–90% of patients develop dyskinesias within 5–10 years. Dyskinesias are more common in younger onset disease (Schrag et al 2003).

There are several clinical risk factors thought to be important in the development of dyskinesias such as duration of disease, severity of disease,

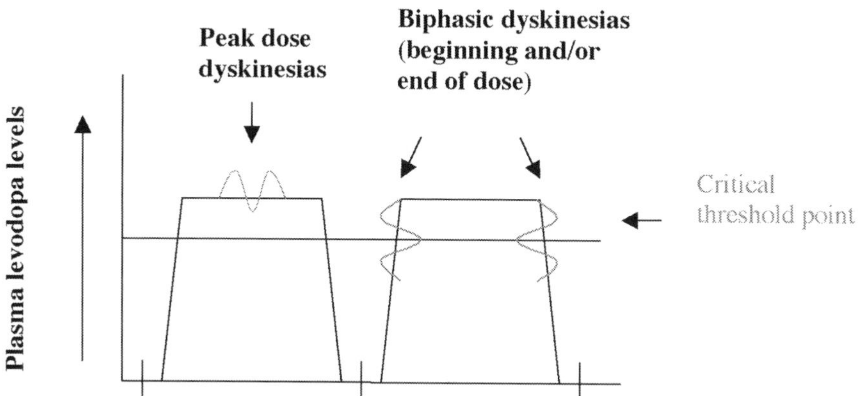

Figure 4.2 The relationship between plasma levodopa levels and peak dose and biphasic dyskinesias.

age of onset of PD and initial levodopa dose (Baas 2000). The exact mechanism responsible for dyskinesias is unclear but theories focus on pulsatile stimulation of DA receptors, supersensitivity of postsynaptic DA receptors and altered glutamatergic activity (Baas 2000).

Dyskinesias can affect any part of the body and can vary in severity. When mild, they may be localized to one part of the body such as a shoulder or a foot and the patient may be unaware of the involuntary movements. However, they can also be generalized, affecting many body parts (face, neck, trunk, arms and legs). Occasionally dyskinesias can be severe (particularly in young-onset disease) and the patient may be unable to perform any purposeful motor tasks. During episodes of severe dyskinesias some patients opt to sit or lie on the floor as they cannot safely sit in a chair or stand.

Most patients will not attempt to undertake certain activities such as climbing stairs or using machinery when moderately or severely dyskinetic. The occupational therapist (OT) is best placed to offer individual advice about home safety issues and provide advice about appropriate aids to promote independence.

As the disease advances, the threshold for producing dyskinesias lowers but the threshold for switching the patient 'on' stays the same (Mouradian et al 1989). This often results in the patient experiencing dyskinesias during all of their 'on' time. Some patients find this too distressing and prefer to spend more time 'off', while others prefer better motor control and are not deterred by their involuntary movements. The severity of dyskinesias often increases during periods of intense concentration, or when the patient is stressed or anxious (Alder 2002).

Prolonged bouts of dyskinesias can be unpleasant and exhausting. Some patients sweat profusely when dyskinetic so a refreshing wash or shower, change of clothes and fluids should be offered once the dyskinesias have subsided. Many patients who experience moderate to severe dyskinesias tend to be underweight. It is unclear whether this is due to the increased energy expenditure associated with the involuntary movements or simply due to the disease symptoms limiting food intake (Cushing et al 2002). Any patients suspected of being underweight should be referred to their local dietician who is best placed to assess nutritional needs and offer expert advice about dietary intake.

Dyskinesias can have a huge impact on patients' day-to-day lives. Simple pleasures, such as going to the cinema or theatre or going out for a meal, may become impossible as many patients fear that their involuntary movements will be disturbing to others around them. Again, the OT can offer practical advice regarding recreational and social activities.

Management of dyskinesias

Dyskinesias are often difficult to manage. It is vital to differentiate between biphasic and peak-dose as the management of each is different. Peak-dose dykinesias may resolve with a reduction of DA-ergic medication (Stocchi et al 1997; Olanow et al 2001) but this may result in the patient having more 'off' time which might not be acceptable to the individual. Biphasic dyskinesias may respond to an increase in DA-ergic medication, or taking doses closer together. Continuous infusion of apomorphine during waking hours can also help to reduce the severity and frequency of dyskinesias (Colzi et al 1998). Moderate to severe dyskinesias may also be palliated by neurosurgical procedures (see Chapter 6).

The drug amantadine has recently been found to have a mild to moderate antidyskinetic effect (Verhagen et al 1998; Paci et al 2001). Amantadine has various sites of action within the brain but the antidyskinetic effect is thought to be mediated by the inhibition of NMDA receptors and the beneficial effect of this drug is often maintained for more than 1 year (Metman et al 1999).

Dystonia

Dystonia is the term given to abnormal and sustained posturing. It commonly affects the feet, toes and neck but can affect any part of the body. Dystonia predominantly occurs in the 'off' state but can occasionally occur as a peak-dose effect (Poewe 1994). Dystonia often occurs in the early hours of the morning, several hours after the last dose of medication, and is a common reason for disturbed sleep in patients with PD (Le Witt 1993). Dystonia can be a distressing symptom, as it is often painful. Foot/toe dystonia can result in the patient having difficulty with footwear and can affect walking.

Management of dystonia

Some patients find massaging the part of the body affected by the dystonia helpful, but others find that this aggravates the pain. 'Off' period dystonia may benefit from treatment strategies that improve 'on' time. Intermittent injections of apomorphine are often helpful to relieve painful 'off' period dystonia (Lees 1993).

Freezing

Freezing tends to be a later feature of PD (Fahn 1995) and can occur in both the 'on' and the 'off' state. Step hesitation is the most common form of freezing; the patient tries to walk but their feet remain as if stuck to the floor. Freezing episodes are usually transient and predominantly occur in confined spaces (e.g. doorways) and when turning. Freezing can also be brought on by sudden sensory input such as a startle or suddenly encountering an obstacle in one's path (Fahn 1995). Freezing episodes can be extremely disabling because of their unpredictable nature and can often result in the patient stumbling and falling. Many also find freezing episodes embarrassing.

Management of freezing

The management of freezing episodes is challenging. It is important to ascertain whether the patient is experiencing 'on' or 'off' period freezing. 'Off' period freezing typically responds to levodopa therapy but this usually worsens 'on' period freezing (Fahn 1995). Dopamine depletion is implicated in 'off' period freezing whereas 'on' period freezing is ill understood. All patients should be offered practical advice/tips on how to avoid or overcome freezing episodes (see Table 4.1).

Table 4.1 Practical advice on how to avoid or overcome freezing episodes

- Patients should avoid doing two things at once, such as walking and talking
- Patients should be given plenty of time to overcome their freezing and should not be rushed as this often worsens the freezing
- Many patients use visual, auditory or internal cues to help them overcome freezing episodes
- Patients who experience freezing episodes may benefit from the input of a physiotherapist
- The patient's home environment can influence freezing; low furniture and cluttered rooms can increase the frequency of freezing. The patient might benefit from contact with an OT who can give advice on the home environment (Robertson et al 2001)

Useful cues

Many patients use a variety of different visual, auditory or internal cues to help them overcome freezing episodes. Cues tend to be quite individual and patients should be encouraged to experiment with different cues to establish which is useful for them. The underlying mechanism for cues being beneficial is still poorly understood.

- *Verbal or auditory cues*: a common auditory cue is to use counting. The patient counts from one to three and tries to walk on the count of three. Others may sing and use rhythm to help them initiate movement
- *Visual cues*: these include putting something on the floor in front of the patient, such as another person's foot or a piece of paper, and then asking the patient to try to walk over the object. Patients who regularly experience freezing episodes may opt to put down sticky tape on the floor in areas where they frequently freeze, e.g. doorways, so that they can use the visual lines to prevent or overcome freezing. Other patients also adapt walking sticks (sometimes referred to as an inverse walking stick). A slat of wood or piece of plastic is attached to the bottom of the stick, at right angles. When the patient experiences a freezing episode the stick is placed in front of the foot and the patient uses this as a visual cue and steps over it

Unpredictable 'on/off' fluctuations

Most patients experience predictable end-of-dose 'off' periods and their 'on' and 'off' periods are related to the timing of their DA-ergic medication. However, as the disease progresses some patients may start to experience unpredictable 'off' periods that do not follow levodopa dose cycles. Unpredictable 'off' periods can be difficult to manage medically and can be devastating for patients and their carers as it becomes difficult to plan their day's activities with any certainty.

The pharmacokinetics of unpredictable 'off' periods is somewhat complex, but essentially any factor which reduces levodopa absorption from the gut may result in suboptimal plasma levodopa levels. Lower peak plasma concentrations of levodopa cause reduced clinical effectiveness of levodopa (Hardoff et al 2001). The critical threshold point (Figure 4.1) required to switch the patient 'on' may not be reached and this may result in a 'dose failure'. Alternatively, there may be a time delay in reaching the threshold point ('delayed-on').

Levodopa absorption

There are two main factors which influence levodopa absorption: gastric emptying and competition with foods at the absorption sites.

Gastric factors

Levodopa is absorbed in the duodenum and jejunum and therefore the rate of stomach emptying is an important factor affecting the rate of absorption of levodopa from the gastrointestinal tract. A variety of factors can slow gastric emptying:

- The rate of gastric emptying is slower in patients with advanced disease (Djaldetti et al 1996)
- Food in the stomach delays gastric emptying (Kelly 1981)
- Constipation can delay gastric emptying through the cologastric reflex (Bojo and Cassuto 1992)

Competition with foods

Levodopa is absorbed in the small intestine and uses a saturable carrier transport system for transfer across the intestinal mucosa. Large neutral amino acids are absorbed into the blood stream using the same transport system, so a high-protein diet might reduce levodopa absorption (Nutt et al 1984). The intestinal transporters have a high capacity for large amino acids, so competition between levodopa and dietary protein is not usually a problem (Stocchi et al 1997). However, the large neutral amino acid transporters within the blood–brain barrier have a low capacity. They are nearly saturated by normal levels of plasma amino acids, so a high-protein meal can reduce the entry of levodopa into the brain (Stocchi et al 1997).

Management of unpredictable 'on/off' fluctuations

Management of unpredictable 'on/off' fluctuations is extremely difficult. The patient and carer should be made aware of the various factors which can influence levodopa levels. The nurse is in an ideal situation to offer practical advice and information about these factors. See Table 4.2.

Table 4.2 Practical advice for managing unpredictable 'on/off' periods

Patients should:

- Complete an 'on/off' chart for a few days – this might illustrate the reason for the unpredictable 'off', e.g. meal times
- Take levodopa preparations before meals and not with or after food (Stocchi et al 1997) as this might be associated with delayed gastric emptying and this will consequently delay levodopa absorption
- Take levodopa preparations with a large glass of water as this will help flush the medication out of the stomach into the small intestine. If only sips of fluid are taken there is a potential for the levodopa tablets or capsules to remain stuck in the stomach for many hours, so delaying absorption (Stocchi et al 1997)

Table 4.2 contd

Patients should:

- Be given information and advice about the role of dietary protein and levodopa entry into the brain
- Be referred to their local dietician for expert advice
- Be given advice on how best to avoid and manage constipation

When patients first start levodopa they are usually told to take it with food as this can help minimize the emetic side effects. However, a tolerance to the emetic properties develops over time so it becomes unnecessary for them to take their levodopa with food (Stocchi et al 1997).

Unfortunately some patients may continue to experience unpredictable 'off' periods, dose failures and delayed 'on' response despite paying close attention to dietary and gastric influences. These patients may benefit from using subcutaneous injections of apomorphine as this drug is not absorbed via the gut (see Chapter 5). The absorption of DA agonists is not influenced by dietary and gastric factors, so these drugs can be taken with food.

Non-motor 'off' period symptoms

Patients can experience a variety of non-motor 'off' period symptoms and these can be classified into three categories: cognitive, autonomic and sensory (Riley and Lang 1993; Hillen and Sage 1996). The more common non-motor 'off' period symptoms are listed in Table 4.3.

Table 4.3 Non-motor 'off' period symptoms

Cognitive changes	Autonomic symptoms	Sensory symptoms
Anxiety	Sweating	Pins and needles
Panic attacks	Feeling hot or cold	Pain
Depression	Bladder dysfunction	Internal tremor
Apathy	(usually urinary urgency)	Dyspnoea
	Abdominal pain	

Non-motor 'off' period symptoms are thought to be experienced by about 60% of patients who have motor fluctuations (Raudino 2001). Usually these symptoms are mild and not problematic but occasionally they can be debilitating and distressing. 'Off' period anxiety and panic attacks can be particularly distressing and, in some cases, patients even have the feeling that they are going to die (Hillen and Sage 1996).

Management of non-motor 'off' periods

It can be helpful to ask patients to complete an 'on/off' chart and to document the time of day that they experience symptoms. This can help to demonstrate whether the patient's symptoms are only occurring during the 'off' period state. If there is no obvious relationship between symptoms and 'off' state then other causes for these symptoms should be investigated. Treatment strategies should be aimed at reducing 'off' time but patients and carers should also be made aware of the cause of these symptoms and the relationship with the patient's medication.

The use of 'on/off' charts

'On/off' charts can be useful in clinical practice as they can help to illustrate the patient's response to medication throughout the day and therefore help to evaluate the effectiveness of the drug regimen. There are several different types of charts available. Simple 'on/off' charts indicate the amount of time the patient spends in the 'on' and the 'off' state, whereas more detailed charts provide information about dyskinesias, severity of symptoms and frequency of freezing.

Ideally patients should complete their own chart but this is not always possible because of handwriting difficulties or cognitive impairment. The person completing the chart should be given clear instruction how to do so, as completion and accuracy of 'on/off' charts are notoriously poor. Many patients, nurses and other healthcare professionals often become confused about the terminology of the various motor fluctuations and use the terms incorrectly. One common mistake is to mix up tremor and dyskinesias. An accurate chart can help clinicians to optimize the patient's medication but an inaccurate 'on/off' chart may have a detrimental effect.

Impact of motor fluctuations

The onset of motor fluctuations marks a crucial point in the management of PD (Dodel et al 2001) and represents a significant source of disability in advanced PD. The treatment options for motor fluctuations have expanded significantly over recent years and several useful algorithms have been developed as treatment guidelines in attempt to avoid the levodopa-related side effects (Jankovic 2000; Olanow et al 2001). Treatment strategies that stimulate DA receptors in a more continuous, less pulsatile manner have recently been highlighted as a way of reducing the risk of developing treatment-associated motor complications (Stocchi 2003; Stocchi and Olanow 2004). However, despite optimal drug treatment, many patients with advanced disease continue to be severely disabled and these patients might benefit from neurosurgical procedures such as deep brain stimulation (see Chapter 6).

With the emergence of motor fluctuations comes the potential for increased impairment, disability and increased carer burden. The patient's ability to work, perform activities of daily living and to participate in social and recreational activities becomes impaired. Several studies have found that health-related quality of life is reduced when motor complications occur (Dodel et al 2001; Keranen et al 2003). Not surprisingly, studies have also found that the quality of life of carers is also reduced (O'Reilly et al 1996). Health economics studies on the cost of PD indicate that healthcare costs increase considerably in patients with motor fluctuations and dyskinesias compared with patients without these symptoms (Dodel et al 2001). There is also a huge hidden cost to the patient in the form of lost wages, informal care-giving and changing roles (Whetten-Goldstein et al 1997).

Treatment strategies should not only be aimed at optimizing medication; patients and their families should be offered education, support and practical advice regarding the management of their individual symptoms. The Parkinson's disease Nurse Specialist (PDNS) is taking on a greater role in the assessment and management of motor fluctuations. The PDNS is ideally placed to coordinate the case management of patients with PD (Noble 1998) and can also ensure that they have appropriate and early access to invaluable resources such as the multidisciplinary team and social services. Caring for patients with motor fluctuations can be challenging but highly rewarding and there is often great scope for innovative practice. Nurses need to have a good understanding of PD and its symptoms in order to meet the ever changing needs of patients with PD.

Key points

- Most patients with Parkinson's disease will develop motor fluctuations within 4–6 years of starting levodopa
- Motor fluctuations can have a profound impact on quality of life
- Treatment strategies should not only be aimed at optimizing medication but patients and their families should be offered education, support and practical advice regarding their individual symptoms
- The PDNS is increasingly taking on a more important role in the assessment and management of motor fluctuations

- It is vital that nurses are able to differentiate between the various motor fluctuations in order properly to assess, plan, implement and evaluate their patient's care

References

Ahlskog J E and Muenter M D (2001) Frequency of levodopa-related dyskinesias and motor fluctuation estimated from cumulative literature. Movement Disorders 16: 448–458.

Alder C H (2002) Relevance of motor complications in Parkinson's disease. Neurology 58: S51–56.

Baas H (2000) Dyskinesias in Parkinson's disease, pathophysiology and clinical risk factors. Journal of Neurology 247(Suppl IV): 12–16.

Bojo L and Cassuto J (1992) Gastric reflex relaxation by colonic distension. Journal of Autonomic Nervous System 38: 57–64.

Colzi A, Turner K and Lees A J (1998) Continuous subcutaneous waking day apomorphine in the long term treatment of levodopa induced interdose dyskinesias in Parkinson's disease. Journal of Neurology, Neurosurgery and Psychiatry 64(5): 573–576.

Cushing M L, Traviss K A and Calne S M (2002) Parkinson's disease: implications for nutritional care. Canadian Journal of Dietetic Practice and Research 63(2): 81–87.

Djaldetti R, Baron J, Ziv I and Melamed E (1996) Gastric emptying in Parkinson's disease; patients with and without response fluctuations. Neurology 46: 1051–1054.

Dodel R C, Berger K and Oertel W H (2001) Health-related quality of life and healthcare utilisation in patients with Parkinson's disease: impact of motor fluctuations and dyskinesias. Pharmacoeconomics 19(10): 1013–1038.

Factor S A (2001) Parkinson's disease: initial treatment with levodopa or dopamine agonists. Current Treatment Options in Neurology 3(6): 479–493.

Fahn S (1995) The freezing phenomenon in Parkinsonism. In: S Fahn, M Hallet, O Lüders and C D Marsden (eds.) Advances in Neurology Volume 67. Philadelphia: Lippincott-Raven pp. 53–64.

Hardoff R, Sula M, Tamir A, Soil A, Front A, Badarna S, Honigman S and Giladi N (2001) Gastric emptying and gastric motility in patients with Parkinson's disease. Movement Disorders 16(6): 1041–1047.

Hillen M E and Sage J I (1996) Nonmotor fluctuations in patients with Parkinson's disease. Neurology 47(5): 1180–1183.

Jankovic J (2000) Parkinson's disease therapy: tailoring choices for early and late disease, young and old patients. Clinical Neuropharmacology 23: 252–261.

Jankovic J (2002) Levodopa strengths and weaknesses. Neurology 58: S19–32.

Katzenschlager R and Lees A J (2003) Treatment of Parkinson's disease: levodopa as the first choice. Journal of Neurology 249(Suppl 2 II): 19–24.

Kelly K A (1981) Motility of the stomach and gastroduodenal junction. In: L R John (ed.) Physiology of the Gastrointestinal Tract. New York: Raven Press pp. 394–410.

Keranen T, Kaakkola S, Sotaniemi K, Laulumaa V, Haapaniemi T, Jolma T, Kola H, Ylikoski A, Satomaa O, Kovanen J, Taimela E, Haapaniemi H and Turunen H, Takala A (2003) Economic burden and quality of life impairment increase with severity of PD. Parkinsonism and Related Disorders 9(3): 163–168.

Lees A J (1993) Dopamine agonists in Parkinson's disease: a look at apomorphine. Fundamental Clinical Pharmacology 7: 121–128.

LeWitt P A (1993) New treatment strategies. Neurology 43(suppl 6)12: S31–37.

Marsden C D and Parkes J D (1977) Success and problems of long-term levodopa therapy in Parkinson's disease. Lancet 1: 345–349.

Metman L V, Del Dotto P, LePoole K, Konitsiotis S, Fang J and Chase T N (1999) Amantadine for levodopa–induced dyskinesias. A 1-year follow-up study. Archives of Neurology 56: 1383–1386.

Mouradian M M, Juncos J L, Fabbrini G and Chase T N (1989) Motor fluctuations in Parkinson's disease. Annals of Neurology 25: 633–634.

Noble C (1998) Parkinson's disease and the role of the nurse specialist. Nursing Standard 92: 46–48.

Nutt J G, Woodward W R, Hammerstad J P, Carter J H and Anderson J L (1984) The 'on-off' phenomenon in Parkinson's disease: relation to levodopa absorption and transport. New England Journal of Medicine 310(8): 483–488.

Olanow C W and Koller W C (1998) An algorithim (decision tree) for the management of Parkinson's dsieaase: treatment guidelines. Neurology 50(3 suppl 3): S1–7.

Olanow C W, Watts R L and Koller W C (2001) An algorithm (decision tree) for the management of Parkinson's disease: treatment guidelines. Neurology 56(11 suppl 5): S1–88.

Paci C, Thomas A and Onofrj M (2001) Amantadine for dyskinesias in patients affected by severe Parkinson's disease. Neurology Science 22: 75–76.

Poewe W H (1994) Clinical aspects of motor fluctuations in Parkinson's disease. Neurology 44(7 suppl 6): S6–9.

O'Reilly F, Finnan F, Allwright S, Smith G D and Ben-Shlomo Y (1996) The effects of caring for a spouse with Parkinson's disease on social, psychological and physical well–being. British Journal of General Practice 46(410): 507–512.

Raudino F (2001) Non motor off in Parkinson's disease. Acta Neurologica Scandinavica 104: 312–315.

Riley D E and Lang A E (1993) The spectrum of levodopa-related fluctuations in Parkinson's disease. Neurology 43: 1459–1464.

Robertson D, Aragon A, Moore G and Whelan L (2001) Rehabilitation and the interdisciplinary team. In: J R Playfer and J V Hindle (eds.) Parkinson's Disease in the Older Patient. London: Arnold pp. 250–272.

Schrag A, Hovris A, Morley D, Quinn N and Jahanshahi M (2003) Young versus older-onset Parkinson's disease and psychosocial consequences. Movement Disorders 18(11): 1250–1256.

Stocchi F (2003) Prevention and treatment of motor fluctuations. Parkinsonism and Related Disorders 9(Suppl 2): S73–81.

Stocchi F, Nordera G and Marsden C D (1997) Strategies for treating patients with advanced Parkinson's disease with disastrous fluctuations and dyskinesias. Clinical Neuropharmacology 20(2): 95–115.

Stocchi F and Olanow C W (2004) Continuous dopaminergic stimulation in early and advanced Parkinson's disease. Neurology 62(1 Suppl 1): S56–63.

Verhagen Metman L , Del Dotto P, LePoole K, van den Munckhof P, Fang J, Mouradian M M and Chase T N (1998) Amantadine as treatment for dyskinesias and motor fluctuations in Parkinson's disease. Neurology 50: 1323–1326.

Whetten-Goldstein K, Sloan F, Kulas E, Cutson T and Schenkman M (1997) The burden of Parkinson's disease on society, family, and the individual. Journal of the American Geriatrics Society 45(7): 844–849.

CHAPTER FIVE
Apomorphine

KIRSTEN TURNER AND LESLEY SWINN

Introduction

Apomorphine is a potent injectable dopamine (DA) agonist with a high affinity to D1- and D2-like receptors and no opiate or addictive properties. Apomorphine cannot be given orally because it undergoes extensive first-pass metabolism to an inactive metabolite. The quality of the response from a single injection of apomorphine is virtually indistinguishable from the response to levodopa (Kempster et al 1990). Its advantages lie in its rapid response and its reliability but it cannot improve upon the best quality of 'on' response achieved with levodopa (Oertel and Quinn 1997). Apomorphine is an effective therapy primarily for patients with Parkinson's disease (PD) who experience a fluctuating and unpredictable motor response to oral antiparkinsonian medications.

History of apomorphine

Apomorphine was first proposed as a treatment for movement disorders 150 years ago but this indication was not investigated until the 1950s (Schwab et al 1951). Struppler and coworkers (1953) were first to report a clear improvement in motor function of parkinsonian symptoms 20 minutes after an injection of apomorphine. Despite its potential as an effective antiparkinsonian treatment, very few studies were undertaken over the following few decades (Cotzias at al 1970). It is likely that the use of apomorphine was limited by a lack of convenient drug administration systems, its short duration of action and its peripheral dopaminergic (DA-ergic) side effects.

There was a resurgence of interest in apomorphine in the 1980s and since then there has been a plethora of studies reporting the clinical effectiveness of apomorphine in treating the symptoms of PD (Chaudhuri et al 1988; Stocchi et al 1993; Colzi et al 1998; Poewe and Wenning 2000;

Manson et al 2002). One of the main reasons for the resurrection of apomorphine was the licence of the antiemetic drug, domperidone. If apomorphine is given without co-administration of domperidone then severe nausea and vomiting are likely. Patients with PD are unable to take other antiemetic medications such as stemetil or metoclopramide as these drugs block central DA receptors and therefore have the potential to reduce motor function.

Use of apomorphine today

It is estimated that 40% of patients with PD will experience fluctuations in motor response within 4–6 years of taking levodopa (Ahlskog and Muenter 2001). The management of motor fluctuations is difficult as disease progression results in a less predictable response to oral medications. Motor fluctuations can have a huge impact on quality of life both for people with PD (Dodel et al 2001; Keranen et al 2003), and their partners or carers (O'Reilly et al 1996). Apomorphine can be a very effective therapy in managing motor fluctuations and thus improving quality of life.

Apomorphine has been licensed since 1993 for use in patients with PD who experience disabling motor fluctuations and who are inadequately controlled by oral antiparkinsonian medications. Routes of administration of apomorphine covered by the licence are:

- Intermittent subcutaneous injection
- Continuous subcutaneous infusion

Other routes of administration, such as rectal (Hughes et al 1991), intranasal (Kleedorfer et al 1991) and sublingual (Durif et al 1993), have been investigated but none of these routes is currently available. Research into effective alternative routes of administration continues.

Intermittent apomorphine

Intermittent apomorphine injections are primarily used as a rescue therapy for disabling 'off' periods, in patients already receiving optimal antiparkinsonian medication (Lees and Turner 2002). Several studies have reported a significant reduction in 'off' time after introducing intermittent subcutaneous apomorphine injections (Kempster et al 1991; Hughes et al 1993; Esteban-Munoz et al 1997). An effective intermittent injection will reverse or avert an 'off' period from occurring and can last for up to 1 hour.

The timing of each injection is crucial if an impending 'off' period is to be averted and patients should be instructed to inject at the first sign that their medication is wearing off. Intermittent injections are usually suitable for patients who have relatively short 'off' periods that occur less than 10 times a day (Hagell and Odin 2001). Patients who experience more frequent and prolonged 'off' periods may be more suited to continuous infusion.

Not all patients are suited to intermittent injections of apomorphine. Patients who are not include those with cognitive impairment and those who experience significant problems with orthostatic hypotension. Practical factors should also be taken in consideration when selecting patients' suitability and these include the patient's or carer's ability and willingness to administer the injections and their ability to recognize 'off' period symptoms. Patients and their carers should be made aware of the potential benefits and side effects of this therapy but at the same time made aware of what it will involve on a day-to-day basis.

Starting intermittent injections of apomorphine

The procedure for initiating intermittent apomorphine may vary according to local guidelines; in most centres the Parkinson's disease Nurse Specialist (PDNS) is responsible for assessing the patient's response to the drug and initiating this therapy. It is vital that patients are assessed correctly to ensure that their response to apomorphine is clearly established. In order to start a patient on subcutaneous intermittent apomorphine it is necessary to carry out an apomorphine challenge. This will allow the following:

- Determination of whether a patient has a positive response to apomorphine
- Establishment of the optimum individual dose of apomorphine, which varies greatly between patients (1–7 mg)
- Observation for possible side effects, including postural hypotension, sedation and hallucinations

A brief outline of the apomorphine challenge procedure is described in Table 5.1.

Table 5.1 Brief outline of the apomorphine challenge procedure

- Patients are pre-treated with domperidone for 3 days before the apomorphine challenge to minimize nausea and vomiting
- An early light breakfast is usually offered as the challenge may take several hours
- The patient must be in an 'off' state before starting the challenge, so the morning PD medication is usually omitted
- The challenge is normally carried out first thing in the morning to avoid unnecessary patient discomfort due to prolonged 'off' time

Table 5.1 contd

- A baseline motor function examination using a clinical assessment tool, such as the Unified Parkinson's Disease Rating Scale, is often performed to provide an objective measurement of the patient's response to consecutive doses of apomorphine
- Single injections of increasing dosages of apomorphine are administered (i.e. 1.5 mg, 3 mg, 5 mg and 7 mg) at 45–60 minute intervals until a response is seen (the patient switches 'on')
- If 7 mg is administered without any effect the patient is usually considered to be a non-responder. However, in rare cases the medical team may consider administering a slightly higher dose
- The patient is closely observed and monitored throughout for any side effects. Blood pressure is usually monitored. The challenge will be stopped if the patient experiences side effects

Once the correct dose of apomorphine has been identified it usually changes very little, if at all, thereafter (Hughes et al 1993).

There are currently two ways to administer intermittent apomorphine:

- Via a pre-filled penject device (APO-goPen®) as shown in Figure 5.1. This system should be discarded every 48 hours, with the needles being changed after each injection. Some patients find this method easier to use and more socially acceptable for carrying and self-injecting in public
- The apomorphine solution is drawn up in an insulin-type syringe. This method requires preparation on a daily basis

Not all patients will need or want to use the pre-filled system and the decision to use the penject device should be made after considering the patient's individual circumstances.

Continuous infusion of apomorphine

Continuous infusion of apomorphine is an effective treatment for patients with advanced disease who experience disabling, frequent and unpredictable motor fluctuations and dyskinesias despite optimal oral DA-ergic treatment. Continuous infusion of apomorphine can be administered in addition to other DA-ergic medications or as a monotherapy. Several studies have reported a significant reduction in patients' 'off' time after initiation of continuous infusion of apomorphine (Chaudhuri et al 1988; Hughes et al 1993; Stocchi et al 1993). Another benefit is that patients can often significantly reduce their daily dosage of levodopa (Chaudhuri et al 1988; Stocchi et al 1993). A more recent finding is that monotherapy infusion of apomorphine not only improves motor fluctuations but also

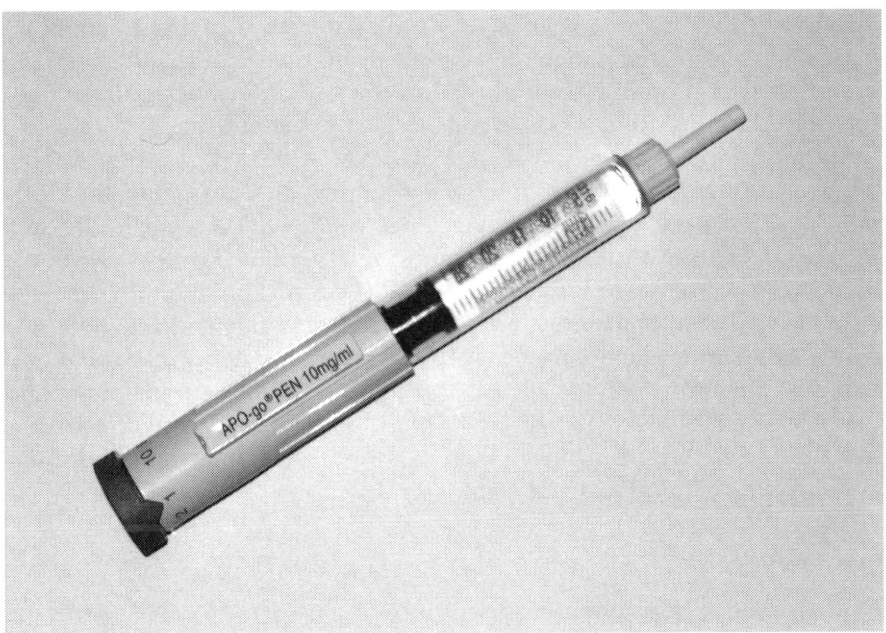

Figure 5.1 Penject device (Courtesy of Britannia Pharmaceuticals Ltd).

has a significant antidyskinetic effect (Colzi et al 1998; Manson et al 2002). Treating patients with continuous infusion of apomorphine is highly effective and in some cases thought to be comparable to neurosurgical procedures (Manson et al 2002).

The aim of continuous infusion in most cases is to provide the patient with more 'on' time and to reduce dyskinesias. It is crucial that patients are realistic about the potential benefits of continuous infusion of apomorphine. Raising expectations too high may result in frustration, low mood and possibly a reduction in quality of life should the therapy fail. Empowering patients and carers so that they are informed before initiating treatment is vital. Information needs to be given in a balanced way so that the benefits and the possible side effects are clearly explained. Patients should be provided with written and video material to support oral information.

Starting on continuous infusion

The procedure for initiating continuous apomorphine will vary according to local guidelines, resources, the philosophy of the medical team and the patient's response to the therapy. Patients need to be admitted to hospital for at least 5 days in order to initiate continuous infusion. In most cases, the aim of the admission is to establish the patient's response to apomorphine and to teach the patient and carer how to manage the infusion. It is very unlikely that optimization of medication will occur during the admission period as this often takes several weeks if not months.

Apomorphine is usually initiated at a low rate (1–2 mg/hour). The dosage is slowly increased as tolerated over several weeks until the optimum dose has been reached or unacceptable side effects are seen. During the period of drug titration it is essential that patients are closely monitored as this will allow early detection of side effects should they occur. The daily dosage of apomorphine varies widely; the current licence recommends a maximum of 100 mg/day although some patients may use more than this. The infusion is usually run during the patient's waking hours but it is occasionally used at night if night-time symptoms are the major problem. There are also a few carefully chosen patients who administer apomorphine continuously, 24 hours per day.

Apomorphine pump

In most cases, apomorphine is administered via the Crono APO-go syringe driver as shown in Figure 5.2. This pump has been specifically designed for the purpose of delivering apomorphine and it is small enough to be easily

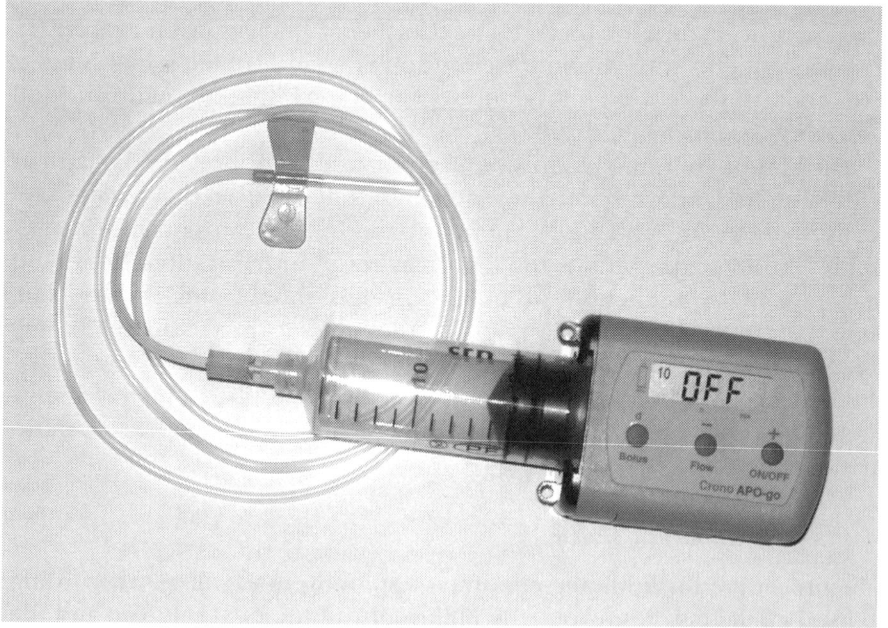

Figure 5.2 APO-go syringe driver (Courtesy of Britannia Pharmaceuticals Ltd).

hidden in a pocket or under a shirt. The pump is only licensed for the use of apomorphine, so many healthcare professionals may be unfamiliar with it. It is relatively easy to use, but nurses must be instructed on how to use it. The PDNS is usually responsible for teaching the hospital and the community nursing staff how to use the pump. Britannia Pharmaceuticals provide a useful video and booklet giving practical information about using the APO-go pump and apomorphine to healthcare professionals.

Although setting up an apomorphine infusion may be relatively simple for health professionals, it may be a daunting prospect for patients and carers. Patients are encouraged to be independent with the administration of the infusion, and a recent study by Manson and others (2002) found that there was a higher rate of success with apomorphine therapy if patients were able to manage the treatment independently or with the help of their caregiver. It is important that patients are aware that they will be supported by their local district nursing teams once discharged. If the patient is unable or unwilling to take on the responsibility of apomorphine, then a partner or carer is often asked to do so. Undue pressure should not be placed on the carer to accept responsibility: for some, it is too much of a burden and additional stress, and in these cases the district nursing service will take on the responsibility.

Patient education

If patients and their carers opt to take on the responsibility of the apomorphine infusion then it is crucial that they are given adequate education and practical experience of using the pump whilst in hospital. The level and the quality of the education given to patients starting on apomorphine therapy can affect compliance and the success of this treatment. It is well recognized that compliance with medication regimes is improved if patients have been educated about their disease and its treatments (Nyatanga 1997). Patients with inadequate education and support will often discontinue apomorphine within weeks. A few hours each day should be set aside for a person with a good knowledge and understanding of apomorphine to teach the patient and carer. Britannia Pharmaceuticals have developed an informative video and booklet for patients which provide practical information about using APO-go pumps and apomorphine.

Information should be given in a structured manner and not left to chance; it is usually the responsibility of the PDNS to coordinate this process. Although patient education should be flexible and individualized to meet the patient's needs, it is essential that core information is imparted. The aim of the education process is to enable the patient and carer to be confident and competent with all aspects of this therapy. Table 5.2 lists some of the key aims of patient education.

Table 5.2 Key aims of patient education

The patient should:

- Be realistic about the benefits of apomorphine
- Know how to prepare and administer apomorphine
- Be able to identify injection sites. The two main areas are the subcutaneous fat on the lower abdominal wall (below the umbilicus) and the upper outer aspects of the thighs. Injection sites should be rotated daily
- Be aware of the importance of good skin management
- Be fully aware of all the potential side effects of apomorphine and know what to do should they occur
- Be aware of the local policy for discarding sharps
- Be aware how to obtain the various pieces of equipment, e.g. infusion lines, syringes and dressings

Discharging patients on apomorphine

Not all patients are completely confident or competent with apomorphine by the date of discharge and, in these cases, the district nurse will provide ongoing supervision, support and education. It is very important that patients and carers feel and receive adequate support and supervision with apomorphine. Patients must be aware of the various key healthcare professionals involved in their care, know the responsibility of each and know how to contact them if needed.

Excellent discharge planning and effective communication between hospital and community teams are essential with apomorphine. General practitioners (GPs) and district nurses must be aware of their responsibilities and it is good practice for them to have a named person as a point of contact in case they need advice. The district nurses should have had training regarding using the APO-go pump before discharge so that they are able to give the patient supervision and support.

Regular follow-up is essential with apomorphine, and during the first few months of starting apomorphine patients should be reviewed regularly in clinic. On a day-to-day basis it is often the responsibility of the PDNS to offer support and advice to both the patient and the community team. The PDNS is in an ideal position to monitor the patient's response to apomorphine and will alert the medical staff promptly if problems occur.

Potential side effects of apomorphine

Most people with parkinsonism tolerate apomorphine but it is important that patients, their carers and nurses are aware of the potential side effects as this will allow early detection and intervention should they occur. Table 5.3 lists the potential side effects of apomorphine.

Table 5.3 Potential side effects of apomorphine

- Nodule formation at needle or infusion site
- Dyskinesias during 'on' time
- Neuropsychiatric complications – hallucinations, euphoria, increased libido, confusion, personality changes, agitation, restlessness, psychosis, sleep disturbance
- Nausea and vomiting
- Sedation
- Postural instability
- Orthostatic hypotension
- Light-headedness
- Haemolytic anaemia
- Eosinophilia

The patient and carer should be advised to be alert for side effects, especially when medication dosages are being adjusted. Patients, carers and nurses should also be aware that, when spilt on clothes and most surfaces, apomorphine will leave a permanent olive green stain that is almost impossible to remove. Should spillage occur, the surface should be washed immediately. Coomb's-positive haemolytic anaemia is a rare side effect of apomorphine (Colzi et al 1993; Hughes et al 1993) and routine blood checks should be carried out at 3-monthly intervals (full blood count, reticulocyte count and Coombs test) (Lees and Turner 2002).

Skin management

The formation of nodules is a common side effect of apomorphine (Frankel et al 1990; Poewe and Wenning 1993; Colzi et al 1998). Some patients will develop severe itchy nodules within a relatively short time, whereas others will have an unblemished skin after several years of apomorphine use (Manson et al 2002). Nodules are easily felt under the skin and are sometimes associated with skin discolouration and scarring (Figure 5.3).

Biopsies of the nodules suggest that the skin response to apomorphine may be caused by a delayed type-1 hypersensitivity reaction (Acland et al 1998). Various factors are thought to be implicated in the development of nodules, such as the amount and frequency of apomorphine being administered (Hagel and Odin 2001); other factors, such as skin type, insertion technique and the weight of the patient may also be important. Nodule formation usually presents a significant clinical problem in only a minority of cases and rarely leads to the discontinuation of apomorphine (Manson

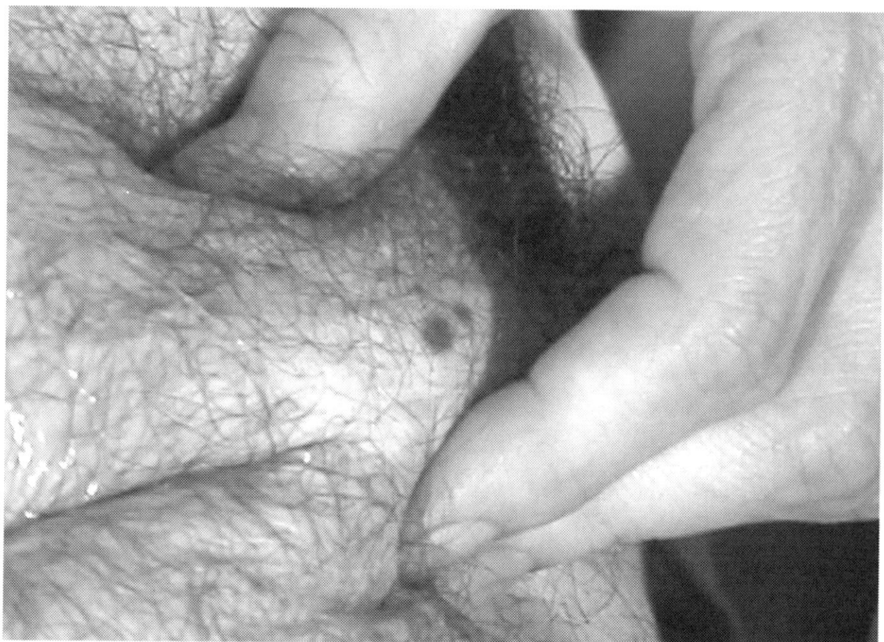

Figure 5.3 Skin discoloration/scarring associated with apomorphine (Courtesy of Britannia Pharmaceuticals Ltd)

et al 2002). However, when nodule formation is severe it may lead to an erratic uptake of apomorphine and consequently may lead to a worsening of symptoms (Turner et al 2001; Manson et al 2002). In addition, the nodules can be very unsightly and painful, and occasionally may become infected.

At present, there are no clear effective strategies to reduce or prevent nodules from occurring (Hagel and Odin 2001). However, anecdotally, local application of ultrasound and silicone gel patches (Turner et al 2001; McGee 2002) have been used with varying effect. More studies are required to gain a better understanding of the various factors implicated in nodule formation and to assess the efficacy of the interventions currently in use. Practical considerations that may help reduce nodule formation are shown in Table 5.4.

Table 5.4 Practical considerations aimed at reducing nodule formation

- Ensure a clean technique
- Good insertion technique is essential. The needle should be inserted at a 45° angle on a horizontal plane when sited in the abdomen and inserted vertically when sited in the thigh. Inserting needle obliquely or vertically in the abdomen can result in trauma, especially in patients with axial dyskinesias

Table 5.4 contd

- Thin patients may not tolerate needle insertion into their thighs as they lack sufficient subcutaneous fat
- It is crucial that the needle site is rotated daily
- Minimize the number of people involved in setting up the infusion. The more people that are involved, the more likely that quality of the insertion technique will vary
- If the needle site becomes red and painful throughout the day it is advisable to remove and reinsert the needle into a new site
- Dilution of the apomorphine with 0.9% normal saline is recommended. If a stronger dilution is used, ulceration of the skin and severe nodule formation occur more commonly (Pollack 1993)
- Patients should be advised to massage the needle site after the needle has been removed. Physiotherapists can teach patients how to perform deep circular massage techniques
- Patients should be advised to seek early medical advice if infection is suspected
- The local PDNS can offer further advice and support regarding skin management

Prescribing issues

In most cases apomorphine is prescribed by GPs following specialist advice from the movement disorder team, although some primary care trusts take the view that apomorphine should only be prescribed by hospital specialists. Whatever the local regulations, the hospital specialists and the primary care team need local agreement and clear guidelines regarding prescribing apomorphine (Hindle and Hindle 2002). As a result, many centres develop shared care guidelines (Turner et al 2001) which reflect local prescribing policy.

Conclusion

Apomorphine is a highly effective treatment for the management of disabling motor fluctuations and has now been used in the UK for more than 15 years. Apomorphine is a valuable part of non-invasive treatment for PD and should be considered before more invasive techniques are tried (Hagell and Odin 2001; Lees 2001). Apomorphine can improve quality of life and keep patients out of costly institutional care for many years (Colzi et al 1998). Key themes to successful outcomes include patient education, ongoing support and follow-up, coordinated care and effective communication between hospital and the primary care team. It is well recognized that success with apomorphine is dependent on the continuing support and advice from PDNS and community nurses.

Key points

- Apomorphine therapy is an effective treatment for patients with advanced PD who experience disabling motor fluctuations despite optimal oral medication
- Key themes to successful outcomes with apomorphine include patient education, coordinated care, ongoing support and follow-up and effective communication between hospital specialists and primary care team
- The PDNS plays a crucial role in initiating, monitoring, educating and supporting patients on apomorphine therapy

Further information

Videos and booklets on apomorphine, and copies of the UCLH shared care guidelines, can be obtained free of charge from: Britannia Pharmaceuticals Ltd, 41–51 Brighton Road, Redhill, Surrey RH1 6YS. Telephone: 01737 773741.

References

Acland K M, Churchyard A, Fletcher C L, Turner K, Lees A and Dowd P M (1998) Panniculitis in association with apomorphine infusion. British Journal of Dermatology 138(3): 480–482.

Ahlskog J E and Muenter M D (2001) Frequency of levodopa-related dyskinesias and motor fluctuation estimated from cumulative literature. Movement Disorders 16: 448–458.

Chaudhuri K R, Critchley P, Abbott R J, Pye I F and Millac P A (1988) Subcutaneous apomorphine for on-off oscillations in Parkinson's disease. Lancet ii(8622): 1260.

Colzi A, Turner K and Lees A J (1998) Continuous subcutaneous waking day apomorphine in the long-term treatment of levodopa-induced interdose dyskinesias in Parkinson's disease. Journal of Neurology, Neurosurgery and Psychiatry 64(5): 573–576.

Cotzias G C, Papavasiliou P S, Tolosa E S, Mendez J S and Bell-Midura M (1970) Similarities between neurologic effects of L-dopa and of apomorphine. New England Journal of Medicine 282(1): 31–32.

Dodel R C, Berger K and Oertel W H (2001) Health-related quality of life and health-care utilisation in patients with Parkinson's disease: impact of motor fluctuations and dyskinesias. Pharmacoeconomics 19(10): 1013–1038.

Durif F, Paire M, Deffond D, Eschalier A, Dordain G, Tournilhac M and Lavarenne J (1993) Relation between clinical efficacy and pharmacokinetic parameters after sub-lingual apomorphine in Parkinson's disease. Clinical Neuropharmacology 16(2):157–166.

Esteban–Munoz J, Marti M J, Marin C and Tolosa E (1997) Long-term treatment with intermittent intranasal or subcutaneous apomorphine in patients with levodopa–related motor fluctuations. Clinical Neuropharmacology 20(3): 245–252.

Frankel J P, Lees A J, Kempster P A and Stern G M (1990) Subcutaneous apomorphine in the treatment of Parkinson's disease. Journal of Neurology, Neurosurgery and Psychiatry 53(2): 96–101.

Hagell P and Odin P (2001) Apomorphine in the treatment of Parkinson's disease. Journal of Neuroscience Nursing 33(1): 21–38.

Hindle C M and Hindle J V (2002) Parkinson's disease and the general practitioner. In: J R Playfer and J V Hindle (eds.) Parkinson's Disease in the Older Patient. London: Arnold pp. 239–249.

Hughes A J, Bishop S, Lees A J, Stern G M, Webster R and Bovingdon M (1991) Rectal apomorphine in Parkinson's disease. Lancet 337(8733): 118.

Hughes A J, Bishop S and Kleedorfer B (1993) Subcutaneous apomorphine in Parkinson's disease: Response to chronic administration for up to five years. Movement Disorders 8(2): 165–170.

Kempster P A, Frankel J P, Stern G M and Lees A J (1990) Comparison of motor response to apomorphine and levodopa in Parkinson's disease. Journal of Neurology, Neurosurgery and Psychiatry 52: 718–723.

Kempster PA, Iansek R and Larmour I. (1991) Intermittent subcutaneous apomorphine injection treatment for Parkinson's disease. Australia and New Zealand Journal of Medicine 21(3): 314–318.

Keranen T, Kaakkola S, Sotaniemi K, Laulumaa V, Haapaniemi T, Jolma T, Kola H, Ylikoski A, Satomaa O, Kovanen J, Taimela E, Haapaniemi H, Turunen H and Takala A (2003) Economic burden and quality of life impairment increase with severity of Parkinson's disease. Parkinsonism and Related Disorders 9(3): 163–168.

Kleedorfer B, Turjanski N, Ryan R, Lees A J, Milroy C and Stern G M (1991) Intranasal apomorphine in Parkinson's disease. Neurology 41(5): 761–762.

Lees, A J (2001) New advances in the management of late stage Parkinson's disease. Review Article. Advances in Clinical Neuroscience and Rehabilitation 1(4): 7–8.

Lees A J and Turner K (2002) Apomorphine for Parkinson's disease. Practical Neurology 2(5): 280–286.

Manson A J, Turner K E and Lees A J (2002) Apomorphine monotherapy in the treatment of refractory motor complications of Parkinson's disease: long-term follow-up study of 64 patients. Movement Disorders 17(6): 1235–1241.

McGee P (2002) Apomorphine treatment: A nurse's perspective. Advances in Clinical Neuroscience and Rehabilitation 2(5): 23–24.

Nyatanga B (1997) Psychosocial theories of patient non-compliance. Professional Nurse 12: 331.

Oertel W H and Quinn N P (1997) Parkinson's disease: Drug therapy. In: N P Quinn (ed) Parkinsonism Clinical Neurology. London: Baillière Tindall pp. 89–108.

Poewe W, Kleedorfer B, Wagner M, Bosch S and Schelosky L (1993) Continuous subcutaneous apomorphine infusions for fluctuating Parkinson's disease. Long-term follow-up in 18 patients. Advances in Neurology 60: 656–9.

Poewe W M D and Wenning G K (2000) Apomorphine: an underutilized therapy for Parkinson's disease. Movement Disorders, 15(5): 789–794.

O'Reilly F, Finnan F, Allwright S, Smith D G and Ben-Shlomo Y (1996) The effects of caring for a spouse with Parkinson's disease on social, psychological and physical well-being. British Journal of General Practice 46(410): 507–512.

Schwab R S, Amador L V and Lettvin J Y (1951) Apomorphine in Parkinson's disease. Transactions of the American Neurological Association 76: 251–253.

Stocchi F, Bramante L, Monge A, Viselli F, Baronti F, Stefano E and Ruggieri S (1993) Apomorphine and lisuride infusion: a comparative chronic study. Advances in Neurology 60: 653–655.

Struppler A and v. Uexkull T (1953) Untersuchungen Uber die Wirkungsweise des Apomorphins auf den Parkinsontremor. Zeitschrift fur Klinische Medizin 152: 46–57.

Turner K, Lees A J and Richardson C (2001) Treatment of Parkinson's Disease with Apomorphine; Shared care edition 4. University College London Hospitals NHS Trust.

CHAPTER SIX
Surgical treatments for Parkinson's disease

CAROLE JOINT AND LESLEY SWINN

Introduction

Pharmacological treatments are the mainstay of therapy for Parkinson's disease (PD) but long-term drug treatment is associated with the emergence of unwanted motor and psychiatric complications. Most patients are reasonably well controlled on medication, but some remain severely disabled with a poor quality of life despite optimal drug treatment. Current medical treatment strategies are aimed at delaying the onset of motor complications and reducing dyskinesias. There has recently been a resurgence of interest in treating PD with neurosurgical procedures and this offers patients further possibilities and hope.

This chapter will discuss a variety of issues related to surgery but the main focus will be on deep brain stimulation (DBS) rather than ablative surgery.

History of surgery in PD

Neurosurgical procedures for the treatment of PD are not new and were commonly performed before levodopa became available in the 1960s when there was no alternative effective treatment. The first surgical approaches targeted the motor cortex and its efferents. The basal ganglia were not targeted until the late 1930s when Russell Meyers began to perform open surgery on the caudate nucleus (Meyers 1958). However, the development of stereotactic surgery (Spiegel and Wycis 1947) led to a surge of interest in applying this new technique to the treatment of PD (Laitinen et al 1992).

Pallidotomies and thalamotomies were extensively performed in the 1950s and 1960s. The thalamus was the most popular target site and Hassler is credited with having carried out the first thalamotomy (Hassler and Riechert 1954). However, with the introduction of levodopa in the 1960s, surgical treatments for PD were almost completely abandoned for all except patients with severe drug-resistant tremor (Lozano et al 1995).

The recent resurgence of interest in surgical procedures is due to limitations in the current medical treatment coupled with advances in the understanding of the basal ganglia motor circuitry and improved targeting techniques.

Targets for PD surgery

Three therapeutic target sites have been identified for the treatment of PD and their anatomical positions within the brain are illustrated in Figure 6.1. They are:

- Thalamus
- Globus pallidus internal segment (GPi)
- Subthalamic nucleus (STN)

Each site may be ablated (destroyed) or stimulated, and surgery can be carried out unilaterally or bilaterally; in practice, few surgeons now perform bilateral ablative surgery and the majority do not create lesions of the STN.

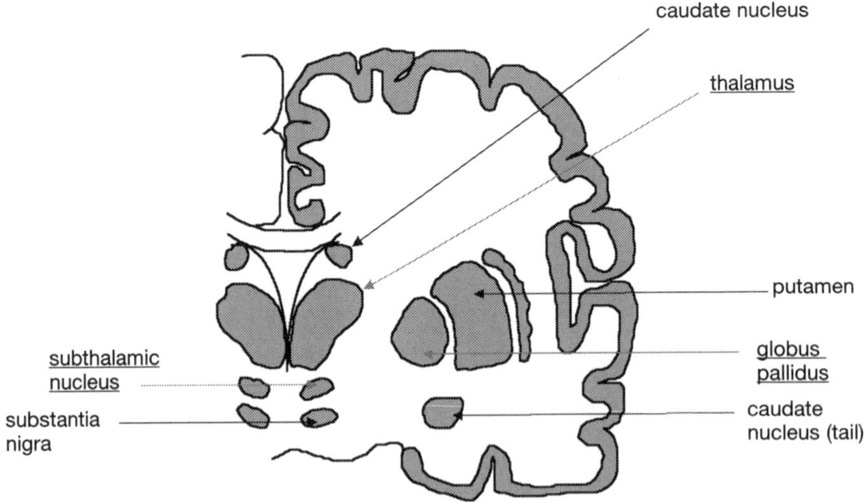

Figure 6.1 Targets for surgical treatments in Parkinson's disease.

Thalamus

The main indication for targeting the thalamus is tremor. The target area within the thalamus is usually the ventral intermediate nucleus (VIM). VIM lesional surgery alleviates contralateral tremor in approximately 70–90% of patients (Tasker 1990). It can also have variable effects on contralateral rigidity and levodopa-induced dyskinesias (Caparros-Lefebvre et al 1993). Thalamic surgery has become increasingly rare except for a minority of patients who are elderly and have tremor-dominant PD (Lang 2000).

Globus pallidus interna (GPi)

Cooper (1956) inadvertently made an important discovery in the physiology of movement disorders when he was performing surgery on a patient who coincidentally had PD. He had to ligate one of the anterior choroidal arteries because of bleeding and found that the patient subsequently showed improvement in the clinical signs of PD on the contralateral side of his body, without any associated motor deficits, despite infarction of the medial pallidum (GPi). Leksell identified the ventral and posterior parts of the GPi as the optimum target sites (Laitinen 2000) and Laitinen and co-workers popularized this procedure (Laitinen et al 1992).

The main reason to target the GPi (lesion or DBS) is to reduce levodopa-induced dyskinesias. Targeting the GPi has a variable effect on parkinsonian symptoms such as rigidity, akinesia and tremor, and this variability is probably due to differences in the precise area of the GPi involved in the procedure. Most clinical studies report a profound reduction of dyskinesias and a reduction in the mean 'off' Unified Parkinson's Disease Rating Scale (UPDRS) motor score (Giller et al 1998; Samuel et al, 1998; Scott et al 1998; Shannon et al 1998).

Pallidal surgery is currently less commonly performed than surgery on the STN. The results of randomized trials reporting a comparison between the two targets, in matched groups of patients, are awaited. Individual patient's symptoms and other factors, such as age, can help functional surgical centres decide which site might be the more appropriate.

Subthalamic nucleus (STN)

The STN is much the most popular target site at present. The idea of targeting this structure came from research performed using monkeys treated with 1-methyl-4-phenyl-1,2,3,6-tetrahydropyridine (MPTP), which showed the STN to be an effective target for the alleviation of PD symptoms (Aziz et al 1992). For many years surgeons were very reluctant to target the STN because of the risk of inducing hemiballismus (a violent, involuntary movement restricted to one side of the body). However, it is now believed that because of the altered physiology in the parkinsonian brain, persistent hemiballismus does not occur although dyskinesias are sometimes seen transiently postoperatively (Guridi and Obeso 2001). A French study was the first to report the benefits of bilateral STN stimulation and reported dramatic improvements in parkinsonian symptoms (Limousin et al 1995; Pollak et al 1996). Bilateral DBS is a very effective treatment for advanced PD and studies have shown that STN surgery is associated with improvements in the UPDRS motor scores in both the 'off' and the 'on' medication state (Deep Brain Stimulation for Parkinson's Disease Study Group 2001). STN surgery also allows significant decreases in levodopa dose in some patients (Limousin et al 1998; Moro et al 1999; Thobois et al 2002).

It is not yet clear whether STN surgery has a direct effect on levodopa-induced dyskinesias, although Benabid et al (2000) reported that it was more difficult to induce dyskinesias in patients following chronic STN stimulation. However, since most patients are able to decrease their daily dosage of levodopa, their dyskinesias are consequently generally reduced.

Surgical techniques

Surgical techniques vary from centre to centre but generally the surgical procedure is carried out in two or three stages:

1. Radiological localization of the target site
2. Physiological localization of the target site (optional)
3. Ablation or stimulation of the target site

Radiological localization

A stereotactic frame is attached to the patient's skull under general or local anaesthestic (Figure 6.2). A stereotactic CT scan and/or MRI scan is performed, usually under a short general anaesthetic, and the reference points within the brain are identified. Some centres use ventriculography for targeting. The position of the target site is calculated using measurements obtained from a stereotactic atlas of the human brain and/or direct visualization of the target structures. In addition, computer software is now available to help in the calculation of the target coordinates by fusing MRI and CT images together in order to obtain a spatially accurate image of the patient's brain.

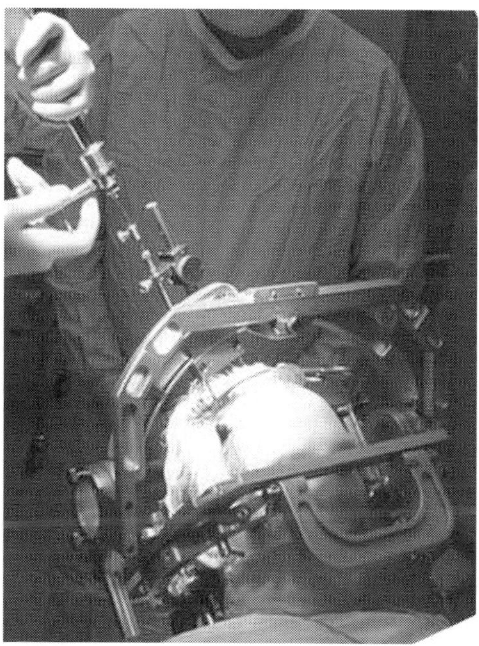

Figure 6.2 Stereotactic frame.

Physiological localization

Surgical centres use a variety of physiological methods to aid final localization of the target site; these may include microelectrode recordings, field potential recordings, clinical assessment during electrical stimulation, somatosensory evoked potentials and electrical stimulation. Not all surgeons use additional physiological techniques as some believe that radiological localization alone is sufficient.

The STN and GPi neuronal cellular activity is distinct from surrounding areas and the surgical team can use this to help them locate the target site with more precision. However, employing physiological methods to aid targeting often prolongs the procedure and can also increase the risk of bleeding (Carroll et al 1998).

Patients are usually awake during the operation if physiological methods are being used, as it is necessary to establish their response to electrical stimulation of the target site. If a general anaesthetic has been given for the scans, it is very important that the anaesthetic technique employed should allow patients to wake up without coughing or vomiting since their head will be fixed to the operating table via the stereotactic frame. It is also necessary to ensure that the anaesthetic does not suppress the patient's parkinsonian signs during the procedure, so all drugs used must be either very short acting or easily reversed. Once the target site is located, the surgeon usually applies high frequency stimulation to the area and this should result in a significant improvement of the patient's contralateral parkinsonian motor signs. Patients should notice a significant improvement within seconds or a few minutes if the electrode is correctly sited.

The brain has no pain receptors so patients will feel little pain during the operation. Local anaesthetic is used for the scalp incision. Patients will be in the 'off' state without medication, so may find it uncomfortable or stressful to lie quietly in the same position for several hours. The stereotactic frame prevents patients from moving their head during the procedure but they will be encouraged to move her legs and arms and helped to adjust their position within this limitation in order to maintain their comfort. The Movement Disorder Nurse, if available, can support and reassure the patient throughout the procedure and assist the neurologist in assessing the patient. If patients wear false teeth, they should bring them to the operating theatre so that they will be able to communicate effectively with the surgical team, and sips of water may be given during the procedure to facilitate speech and maintain comfort for the patient. The anaesthetist will administer pain relief or mild sedatives if the patient is in any discomfort, but again, these must not suppress the PD signs.

Abalation or stimulation of target site

Once the target site has been identified the surgeon will either:

- Create a permanent lesion by heating the tip of a lesioning electrode, or
- Implant the deep brain stimulation (DBS) electrode

If DBS is being used, the stimulation electrode is then replaced by a quadripolar DBS electrode that is firmly anchored to the skull. Some centres externalize the DBS electrodes for a few days in order to test the stimulation and confirm that the patient's parkinsonian symptoms are sufficiently improved before fully implanting the DBS system. Others implant the whole system in a single procedure. In the latter case, the patient will be anaesthetized and the stereotactic frame removed before the leads, extension wires and pulse generator are internalized. The leads and extensions are tunnelled subcutaneously between the scalp and the chest and then connected to the implantable pulse generator as illustrated in Figure 6.3.

The length of the procedure varies considerably, from approximately 2 to 15 hours. Important factors that determine procedure time include the experience of the surgical team, whether physiological methods for targeting are being used, whether bilateral or unilateral surgery is being performed and whether the electrode and battery are being internalized.

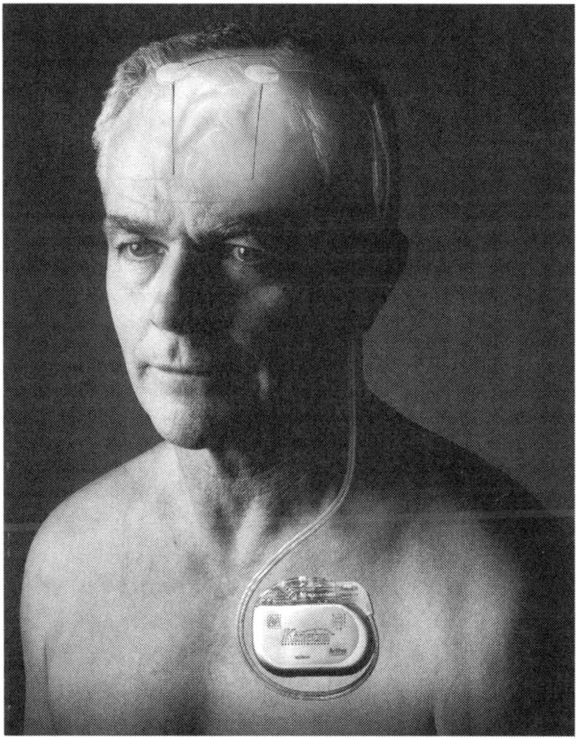

Figure 6.3 The implanted DBS system. (Reproduced with permission of Medtronic UK)

Unilateral or bilateral surgery?

Most surgeons are reluctant to perform bilateral ablative procedures as there is an increased risk of complications, particularly involving speech and cognition (Kumar et al 1998). Unfortunately very few patients with PD have unilateral symptoms. Certainly, bilateral thalamic lesions should not be performed, as the risk of severe speech impairment is extremely high. Bilateral GPi lesions can be safely performed by experienced surgeons (Scott et al 1998) but are rarely carried out now, partly because it is thought that destructive procedures are inadvisable if there is a chance of restorative techniques being available for the patient in the future. Bilateral DBS seems to be associated with a lower risk of morbidity than bilateral lesions (Krack et al 1999) and many now view this as the operation of choice. Some centres still advocate the use of unilateral lesions, generally as a palliative procedure in elderly patients (Gregory 2002) and there will always be some countries in which DBS is too costly to become a mainstream therapy (Green at al 2004).

DBS or lesion?

The advantages and disadvantages of the two techniques are illustrated in Table 6.1.

Table 6.1 Advantages and disadvantages of DBS versus lesion

Advantages	Disadvantages
DBS	
Bilateral surgery possible without increased risk of complications	Costly – bilateral surgery costs in the region of £30,000
A permanent lesion is not created so the procedure is reversible	Battery life is currently only 3–7 years and thus it may need replacement
Stimulation parameters can be adjusted in an attempt to maximize efficacy and minimize adverse effects	Need for regular follow-up and reprogramming
	Hardware-related complications (infection, erosion, breakage of wires)
Lesion	
Cheap	Permanent, although there may be some loss of benefit over time
No maintenance required	Bilateral thalamic lesions not possible, and STN lesions are not recommended
Permanent	Some studies have suggested that bilateral lesions are associated with increased complications, especially those related to speech and cognition

Mechanism of action of DBS

DBS at high frequency probably has an inhibitory effect on the output from the target structures (Benabid et al 1987) but the exact mechanisms that underlie this are not known. The inhibitory activity could be due to membrane hyperpolarization but this may differ depending on the region stimulated (Dostrovsky and Lozano 2002). McIntyre et al (2004) discuss four further hypotheses to explain the mechanism of DBS: depolarization blockade, synaptic inhibition, synaptic depression and stimulation-induced modulation of activity. It is thought that high-frequency stimulation (>50 Hz, and usually 130–180 Hz) mimics the effect of an ablative procedure (Benabid et al 2002). The overall effect, whatever the mechanism, is to 'jam' the output from overactive circuits in the basal ganglia in PD.

Patient selection

Large numbers of patients are now being referred to neurological centres to be considered for surgery for PD. Careful discussions between neurologists and neurosurgeons take place in order to identify potential candidates. The media and internet have helped to improve patient and public awareness of the surgical treatments, especially DBS of the STN, but this can sometimes lead to patients having unrealistic expectations.

Most centres have a rigorous selection process that aims to identify candidates. The following criteria are used:

- Patients who will obtain the greatest benefit from the treatment
- Patients who will maintain this benefit long enough to justify time and money invested
- Patients who are physically, mentally and emotionally able to tolerate all aspects of surgery and postoperative care (Lang and Widner 2002)

A careful medical history should be taken, since some co-existing conditions may preclude surgery. Uncontrolled hypertension, anticoagulant therapy and aspirin are all contraindications to functional surgery and such issues must be addressed, if possible, well in advance of the patient's admission to hospital. For example, it may be possible to stop aspirin treatment, and if so, this should be done 3–4 weeks before surgery.

An important issue to address is at what stage of the disease to consider surgery. This is a difficult and controversial area. Many neurologists believe that undertaking surgery with all its attendant risks is generally not justified in patients with early or mild disease. Patients with more advanced disease and motor complications are generally more suitable candidates because, for them, the probable benefits of surgery will usually outweigh the risks associated with the procedure. If patients are very advanced in their disease, they may become unsuitable candidates for surgery since speech, swallowing and balance are generally not improved by surgery.

During outpatient consultations, patients and their families must be given comprehensive information about the probable benefits and the possible risks of surgery so that they are in a position to make an informed decision about whether they wish to proceed. In any event, it is advisable to allow patients to go home with appropriate written information and a contact number for the movement disorder team in case they have any further questions, before making a final decision about whether to undergo surgery.

Patient assessment and evaluation

An important area within any surgical programme is to establish how to evaluate the effectiveness of the surgical procedure. A useful and widely used protocol for evaluating surgical outcomes is the Core Assessment Program for Surgical Interventional Therapies in Parkinson's Disease (CAPSIT-PD) (Defer et al 1999). This protocol includes recommendations on patient selection, frequency of patient assessment and details of which tests to use to quantify symptoms. Assessment of quality of life should be included in the protocol both before and after surgery.

Such assessments form an important part of the selection process, in terms of whether the patient is likely to benefit from surgery and, if so, which procedure may be the most appropriate. In addition, the time spent in carrying out assessments provides an important opportunity to establish a rapport with patients and to clarify what their expectations of surgery are.

It is important to establish whether a patient has any significant cognitive difficulties, because it is now known that such patients usually do not achieve a good outcome from surgery, and most centres will include detailed neuropsychometry in their preoperative assessment process.

DBS

Complications of DBS

The complications of DBS are similar for all three target sites (thalamus, GPi and STN) and can be categorized into three groups (Olanow et al 2000):

- Those related to the surgical procedure, e.g. haemorrhage, ischaemic lesions and seizures. These can be life threatening
- Those associated with the device, e.g. displacement of the electrode, skin erosion or infection or mechanical problems with the electrical system
- Those caused by the stimulation, e.g. paraesthesia, muscle contractions, pain and abnormal eye movements

The morbidity associated with DBS is generally considered to be less than with ablative surgery (Krack et al 1999).

Programming the stimulator and adjusting medication

Programming the DBS is usually started during the first few days after surgery and the need to adjust medication at this time will depend on which surgical target has been used. The patient who has had thalamic surgery carried out for tremor alone may not have been taking any medication prior to surgery because nothing was effective for their tremor. Those patients who were taking medication will generally continue to do so, often with little change from their preoperative dose (Limousin-Dowsey et al 1999). Pallidal surgery usually requires little or no adjustment of medication postoperatively, although some patients may need to increase their dose of L-dopa if they were undermedicated preoperatively because of disabling dyskinesias. If the patient required apomorphine before pallidal surgery, this is usually no longer needed postoperatively.

STN surgery often allows a substantial reduction in PD medication and this is managed alongside the DBS programming. The aim is to optimize stimulation and supplement as necessary with medication in order to achieve the best control of PD for the patient (Volkmann et al 2001). STN stimulation and PD medication have an additive effect on the control of PD, and dyskinesias may result if medication is not reduced when DBS is commenced. There have been reports of depression and suicide following STN surgery, and this may be due to the reduction in levodopa therapy, or a direct effect of stimulation on the limbic pathways (Krack et al 1998, 2001). Further research is needed in order to clarify this issue.

Sometimes a micro-lesioning effect occurs when the DBS leads are placed, and this may result in significant reduction in the patient's PD signs. In this case, it will normally be necessary to delay the initial titration of DBS until the patient's PD signs have returned. Regardless of when stimulation is started it is usual to have to make several adjustments to the stimulation parameters during the following weeks in order to achieve maximum benefit. Patients should be informed of this at the outset so that they are not disappointed if they feel that the outcome of surgery is not optimal in the early postoperative period. Stimulation parameters are generally fairly stable from about 3 months after surgery.

Side effects of stimulation

There are many possible side effects of stimulation, the commonest being dysarthria and dysaesthesia. Transient dysaesthesia is relatively common during initial titration of the DBS, but usually resolves over a few seconds or with selection of a different electrode contact for stimulation. Stimulation of the STN can occasionally cause transient dyskinesias in the immediate postoperative period but these generally resolve over a period of a few days.

Persistent side effects can be avoided by careful programming of the DBS parameters but, if accompanied by inadequate control of PD symptoms, they may indicate that the position of the DBS lead is sub-optimal.

One of the most frequently occurring adverse effects of chronic stimulation of STN or GPi is weight gain, often of several kilograms (Volkmann et al 2001). This may be an advantage for a patient who was significantly underweight preoperatively, but it can prove quite distressing for some patients and they should be warned of this possibility before surgery.

Nursing care of the patient

Preoperative care

Preoperative care is aimed at ensuring that patients is prepared for surgery both physically and psychologically. Much of the psychological support for patients and their families will be provided by the Movement Disorder or Surgical Parkinson's Disease Nurse Specialist who should also be involved in planning nursing care with the ward nurses. It is important to allow patients to maintain control of their own medication if possible, and a self-medication protocol can ensure safety, although it will usually be necessary to suspend this during the perioperative period.

Perioperative care

Perioperative care firstly involves ensuring that the patient is in the 'off-medication' state and fully prepared for surgery. The patient will need to be 'nil by mouth' because a general anaesthetic is often given at some stage during the procedure, but precise preoperative instructions will vary according to local practice. Functional neurosurgical procedures are usually carried out first thing in the morning in order to prevent the patient from having to remain in the 'off' state for longer than is absolutely necessary. An important part of the role of the Movement Disorder Nurse is to provide nursing care and support for the patient throughout the perioperative period, including the time in the anaesthetic room, operating theatre and recovery area. It is beneficial to the patient to have a familiar person with them, it is valuable in terms of intraoperative assessment, and it is also important for effective communication with the ward staff and the patient's family after the procedure (Joint 1997).

Postoperative care

Postoperative care will vary according to local protocols, but is aimed at early recognition and management of complications following surgery.

Careful observation for neurological deterioration is essential, especially intraoperatively and in the immediate postoperative period, when the risk of intracerebral haemorrhage is at its highest. The patient is usually allowed to get out of bed to use the toilet as necessary once back on the ward, provided that they are neurologically stable. Mobilization is encouraged as soon as the patient feels able.

Wound care is important since the consequences of infection can be very serious, both in terms of the patient's safety and also because it may necessitate removal of the DBS system. It is usual to give intraoperative and postoperative antibiotics as prophylaxis.

Discharge from hospital and follow-up

The time-scale for discharge from hospital is varied and will depend on many factors, including the following:

- Satisfactory postoperative recovery
- Titration of DBS
- Titration of medication
- Distance patient has to travel
- Home circumstances

Initial follow-up is usually at about 4–6 weeks after surgery, primarily to ensure that the wounds have healed and to assess the degree of control of symptoms. The DBS parameters and medication may be adjusted at this time and subsequent appointments will be made for titration of the DBS according to the patient's response. Contact by telephone can be extremely helpful during this time and may prevent patients from travelling to the hospital unnecessarily, as many issues can be resolved by providing explanation and reassurance for patients and their family.

Patient and family education

Patient and family education should be started at the time of the first outpatient consultation and continued during the preoperative and postoperative period. Information should be provided in both verbal and written format and be aimed at ensuring that all the patient's questions are answered in a way that they can understand.

Patients may be given a hand-held programmer that can allow them some control over their DBS parameters within limits that are pre-set by the clinician. It can also allow them to check whether the pulse generator battery is 'on' or 'off' or reaching the end of its life. Some patients may have an old-style pulse generator implanted that may be switched on or off by means of a magnet that the patient is given, but the patient cannot adjust stimulation settings with this system.

The company that manufactures the DBS system has produced some literature which includes details of medical treatments that must be avoided by patients with a DBS implanted. It also contains some advice about general domestic appliances that may interfere with the device, but this needs to be supplemented by additional information from the clinicians and should include advice about lifestyle implications of DBS.

N.B. There is a specific warning that short-wave diathermy and ultrasound diathermy treatments are absolutely contraindicated for patients with DBS.

There are clearly some lifestyle implications for patients once they have a DBS system implanted. Since the aim of surgery is to improve the quality of life for patients and their families, they should be encouraged to lead as full a life as possible. Many non-contact sports, hobbies and leisure activities are permissible and should be encouraged if the patients wish and are able to participate. Advice about specific activities can be obtained from the Movement Disorder Team.

Conclusions

Surgical procedures for PD have re-emerged as an option for patients and can offer hope of an improved quality of life for some. This chapter has discussed the selection, assessment and management of these patients with an emphasis on the multidisciplinary nature of care. Current surgical treatments are only able to modify symptoms in the patient with PD. Most clinicians involved in these therapies regard the future as being in restorative procedures, perhaps using growth factors or stem cells, and much research is currently being undertaken in these areas. Further insight into these can be found in Chapter 16.

It is important that centres embarking on a programme of surgical treatments for PD and other movement disorders have access to appropriate specialist staff and facilities to ensure the best care for their patients before, during and after surgery. Such expertise and equipment will not be available in every hospital and it is therefore beneficial for patients, and more cost effective, to concentrate these services in a fairly small number of centres. The disadvantage of this will be that patients often have to travel some distance from their homes for treatment; it is therefore crucial that communication between the specialist staff in hospital and the primary care team is both timely and comprehensive so that those caring for patients in the community can do so effectively. A specialist nurse working within the multidisciplinary team in the hospital can provide an invaluable link in this area. This is an exciting speciality to work within and nurses caring for patients with PD should embrace these developments.

Key points

- Surgery for Parkinson's disease is not new
- Current target sites include the thalamus, the globus pallidus and the subthalamic nucleus
- Surgical techniques vary but their common aim is to modify the abnormal neuronal activity within the basal ganglia and therefore improve the cardinal symptoms of the disease
- Patients and their families need to be fully informed about the procedure and its implications so that they can make informed decisions
- The provision of specialist nursing will help patients and their families to cope with the preoperative assessments, surgical procedure and postoperative phases

References

Aziz T Z, Peggs D, Agarwal E, Sambrook M A and Crossman A R (1992) Subthalamic nucleotomy alleviates parkinsonism in the 1-methyl-4-phenyl-1,2,3,6-tetrahydropyridine (MPTP)-exposed primate. British Journal of Neurosurgery 6: 575–582.

Benabid A L, Pollak P, Louveau A, Henry S and de Rougemont J (1987) Combined (thalamotomy and stimulation) stereotactic surgery of the VIM thalamic nucleus for bilateral Parkinson disease. Applied Neurophysiology 50: 344–346.

Benabid A, Koudsie A, Benazzouz A, Fraix V, Ashraf A, Le Bas J F, Chabardes S and Pollak P (2000) Subthalamic stimulation for Parkinson's disease. Archives of Medical Research 31: 282–289.

Benabid A L, Benazzous A and Pollack P (2002) Mechanisms of deep brain stimulation. Movement Disorders 17(suppl 3): S73–74.

Caparros–Lefebvre D, Blond S, Vermersch P, Pecheux N, Guieu J D and Petit H (1993) Chronic thalamic stimulation improves tremor and levodopa induced dyskinesias in Parkinson's disease. Journal of Neurology, Neurosurgery and Psychiatry 56: 268–273.

Carroll C, Scott R, Davies L E and Aziz T (1998) The pallidotomy debate. British Journal of Neurosurgery 12(2): 146–150.

Cooper I S (1956) The Neurosurgical Alleviation of Parkinsonism. Springfield, Illinois: Charles C Thomas.

Deep Brain Stimulation for Parkinson's Disease Study Group (2001) Deep-brain stimulation of the subthalamic nucleus or the pars interna of the globus pallidus in Parkinson's disease. New England Journal of Medicine 345:956–963.

Defer G L, Widner H, Marie R M, Remy P and Levivier M (1999) Core assessment program for surgical interventional therapies in Parkinson's disease (CAPSIT-PD). Movement Disorders 14: 572–584.

Dostrovsky J O and Lozano A M (2002) Mechanisms of deep brain stimulation. Movement Disorders 17(suppl 3) S63–68.

Giller C A, Dewey R B, Ginsburg M I, Mendelsohn D B and Berk A M (1998) Stereotactic pallidotomy and thalamotomy using individual variations of anatomic landmarks for localization. Neurosurgery 42: 56–65.

Green A, MacIntosh E, Joint C, Sethi H, Bain P and Aziz T (2004) Cost analysis of unilateral and bilateral pallidotomy for Parkinson's disease. Journal of Clinical Neuroscience 11(8): 829–834.

Gregory R (2002) Surgery for movement disorders. Journal of Neurology, Neurosurgery and Psychiatry 72(Suppl 1): I32–35.

Guridi J and Obeso J A (2001) The subthalamic nucleus, hemiballismus and Parkinson's disease: reappraisal of a neurosurgical dogma. Brain 124: 5–19.

Hassler R and Riechert T (1954) Indikationen und Lokalisations-methode der gezielten Hirnoperationenen. Nervenarzt 25: 441–447.

Joint C (1997) A multi-disciplinary approach to pallidotomy and thalamotomy in the management of Parkinson's disease. British Journal of Theatre Nursing 7: 5–8.

Krack P, Hamel W, Mehdorn H M and Deuschl G (1999) Surgical treatment of Parkinson's disease. Current Opinion in Neurology 12: 417–425.

Krack P, Pollak P, Limousin P, Hoffmann D, Xie J, Benazzouz A and Benabid A L (1998) Subthalamic nucleus or internal pallidal stimulation in young onset Parkinson's disease. Brain 121(3): 451–457.

Krack P, Ardouin C, Funkiewiez A, Caputo E, Benazzouz A, Benabid A L and Pollack P (2001) What is the influence of STN stimulation on the limbic loop? In: K Kultas-Ilinsky and I A Ilinsky (eds.) Basal Ganglia and Thalamus in Health and Movement Disorders. New York: Kluwer Academic/Plenum Publishers pp. 333–340.

Kumar R, Lozano A M, Montgomery E and Lang A E (1998) Pallidotomy and deep brain stimulation of the pallidum and subthalamic nucleus in advanced Parkinson's disease. Movement Disorders 13(suppl 1): S73–82.

Laitinen L V (2000) Leksell's unpublished pallidotomies of 1958–1962. Stereotactic and Functional Neurosurgery 74: 1–10.

Laitinen L V, Bergenheim A T and Hariz M I (1992) Leksell's posteroventral pallidotomy in the treatment of Parkinson's disease. Journal of Neurosurgery 76: 53–61.

Lang A E (2000) Surgery for Parkinson's disease. A critical evaluation of the state of the art. Archives of Neurology 57: 1118–1125.

Lang A E and Widner H (2002) Deep brain stimulation for Parkinson's disease: Selection and evaluation. Movement Disorders 17(suppl 3): S94–101.

Limousin P, Pollak P, Benazzouz A, Hoffmann D, Le Bas J F, Brousolle E and Perrett J E (1995) Effect on parkinsonian signs and symptoms of bilateral subthalamic nucleus stimulation. Lancet 345: 91–95.

Limousin P, Krack P, Pollak P, Benazzouz A, Ardouin C, Hoffmann D and Benabid A L (1998) Electrical stimulation of the subthalamic nucleus in advanced Parkinson's disease. New England Journal of Medicine 339: 1105–1111.

Limousin–Dowesy P, Pollack P, Van Blercom N, Krack P, Benazzouz A and Benabid A L (1999) Thalamic, subthalamic nucleus and internal pallidum stimulation in Parkinson's disease. Journal of Neurology 246(Suppl 2): 42–45.

Lozano A M, Lang A E, Galvez-Jimenez N , Miyasaki J, Duff J, Hutchinson W D and Dostrovsky J O (1995) Effect of GPi on motor function in Parkinson's disease. Lancet 346: 1383–1387.

McIntyre C C, Savasta M, Walter B L and Vitek J L (2004) How does deep brain stimulation work? Present understanding and future questions. Journal of Clinical Neurophysiology 21(1): 40–50.

Moro E, Scerrati M, Romito L M, Roselli R, Tonali P and Albanese A (1999) Chronic subthalamic nucleus stimulation reduces medication requirements in Parkinson's disease. Neurology 53:85–90.

Meyers R (1958) Historical background and personal experiences in the surgical relief of hyperkinesias and hypertonus. In: W Fields (ed.) Pathogenesis and Treatment of Parkinsonism. Springfield, Illinois: Charles C Thomas pp. 229–270.

Olanow C W, Brin M F and Obeso J A (2000) The role of deep brain stimulation as a surgical treatment for Parkinson's disease. Neurology 55: S60–66.

Pollak P, Benabid A L, Limousin P, Benazzouz A, Hoffmann D, Lebas J F and Perret J (1996) Subthalamic nucleus stimulation alleviates akinesia and rigidity in parkinsonian patients. Advances in Neurology 69: 591–594.

Samuel M, Caputo E, Brooks D J (1998) A study of medial pallidotomy for Parkinson's disease: clinical outcome, MRI location and complications. Brain 121: 59–75.

Scott R, Gregory R, Hines N, Carroll C, Hyman N, Papanasstasiou V, Leather C, Rowe J, Silburn P and Aziz T (1998) Neuropsychological, neurological and functional outcome following pallidotomy for Parkinson's disease. A consecutive series of eight simultaneous bilateral and 12 unilateral procedures. Brain 121: 659–675.

Shannon K M, Penn R D, Kroin J S (1998) A study of medial pallidotomy for Parkinson's disease. Efficacy and adverse effects at 6 months in 26 patients. Neurology 50: 434–438.

Spiegel E A and Wycis H T (1947) Stereotaxic apparatus for operations on the human brain. Science 106: 349–350 (Abstract).

Tasker R R (1990) Thalamotomy. Neurosurgery Clinics of North America 1: 841–864.

Thobois S, Mertens P, Guenot M, Hermier M, Mollion H, Bouvard M, Chazot G, Brousolle E and Sindou M (2002) Subthalamic nucleus stimulation in Parkinson's disease: clinical evaluation of 18 patients. Journal of Neurology 249(5): 529–534.

Volkmann J, Fogel W and Krack P (2001) Stimulation of the subthalamic nucleus for Parkinson's disease. Medtronic Ltd, UK.

CHAPTER SEVEN
Bladder, bowel and sexual function in Parkinson's disease

COLLETTE HASLAM AND RANAN DASGUPTA

Introduction

Bladder, bowel and sexual problems can be very embarrassing and difficult to talk about. Many patients will put up with what they see as their problem and in fact many go to great lengths to conceal problems. This is a great pity as, today, there is much that can be done to help patients to manage such problems. It is important that nurses have an understanding of the assessment and management of pelvic organ disorders so that they can offer appropriate care.

This chapter will address bladder, bowel and sexual dysfunction in Parkinson's disease (PD), covering symptoms, investigations and practical management.

Bladder function

> In health and continence the decision when to void is determined by the perceived state of bladder fullness together with an assessment of the social appropriateness to do so (Fowler, 1999).

We are not born with control of our bladder function; it is something we acquire as the central nervous system matures. This control is extremely complex and therefore it is not surprising that dysfunction occurs in neurological disease. Bladder control is maintained by a series of nerve pathways between the brain and the spinal cord which is believed to maintain a reciprocal relationship between the function of the bladder and that of the sphincter outlet during the two phases of storage and voiding (Craggs and Vaizey 1999).

Bladder dysfunction in Parkinson's disease

Bladder problems are not inevitable with PD, although many patients do have some form of bladder dysfunction, particularly in the advanced stages of the disease. Sakakibara et al (2001) found that PD patients with urinary dysfunction had a higher Unified Parkinson's Disease Rating Scale score and higher Hoehn–Yahr grade; this finding suggests that bladder dysfunction in PD is related to disease progression. Neuronal degeneration in the areas of the brain that control micturition is responsible for a variety of bladder symptoms in patients with PD. It has been suggested that the basal ganglia have an inhibitory affect on the micturition reflex in normal circumstances and, with the cell loss in the substantia nigra that occurs in PD, bladder overactivity occurs (Chandiramani and Fowler 1999).

Whilst it is generally accepted that detrusor overactivity is the commonest cause of urinary symptoms in patients with PD, it has also been suggested that symptoms may also be caused by bradykinesia of the bladder sphincter (a failure to relax when voiding) (Araki and Kuno 2000). Some male patients with PD may also have additional benign prostatic hyperplasia, contributing to symptoms of voiding obstruction, such as hesitancy or poor flow (Chandiramani and Fowler 1999). Urinary symptoms are often worse in the 'off' state (Raudino 2001). These symptoms can include frequency, urgency, urge incontinence and those of incomplete emptying.

Definition of terms

These definitions are taken from the report from the Standardization Subcommittee of the International Continence Society (Abrams et al 2002).

- Urgency: a sudden compelling desire to pass urine, which is difficult to defer
- Urge urinary incontinence: any involuntary leakage accompanied by or immediately preceded by urgency
- Increased daytime frequency: the patient considers that he or she voids too often by day
- Nocturia: the individual has to wake at night one or more times to void
- Hesitancy: difficulty in initiating micturition, resulting in a delay in the onset of voiding after the individual is ready to pass

Impact of bladder symptoms on the quality of life of patients and their carers

Bladder symptoms have been found to have an impact on patients' quality of life (Grimby et al 1993). Symptoms of bladder dysfunction are often exacerbated by patients' poor neurological status, causing, for example, a delay in getting to the toilet due to reduced mobility and difficulty removing the necessary clothing once there. Some patients avoid going outside or socializing because of their failure to cope.

One study by Lees et al (1988) explored night-time problems in 220 patients with PD and found that one third had to get up three or more times to pass urine. This does not only affects patients; the disruption caused to their partners' night sleep can have a profound effect on their partners' quality of life.

Assessing bladder function

The nurse is in the ideal position to identify and assess bladder problems. The nurse should note:

- History of lower urinary tract symptoms, i.e. frequency, urgency, hesitancy, nocturia and incontinence. A urine sample (dipstick) should be checked for leucocytes and nitrites as many patients have underlying urinary tract infections that may exacerbate their symptoms
- Onset and duration of symptoms
- Amount and type of fluid intake. It is usually recommended that the patient should aim to drink 1.5–2 litres of fluid in 24 hours. Caffeinated drinks such as coffee, tea and colas can stimulate the detrusor muscle and so worsen bladder symptoms
- Past medical history, including obstetric, gynaecological and urological history
- Medication (this should include PD treatment that could have anticholinergic side effects)
- Mobility and dexterity
  - Can the patient get to the toilet independently, both day and night?
  - Can the patient manage to adjust clothing for the toilet?
- Psychological issues i.e. patient's awareness of the problem, attitude, motivation and mental impairment
- Carer involvement. How much assistance does the patient require for the following?
  - Getting to and from the toilet
  - Getting in and out of bed
  - Maintaining adequate diet and fluids
  - Washing and dressing
  - Using appliances

It is important to obtain a baseline of the patient's continence status before instigating treatment or management. With thought and patience nurses may be able to offer patients practical advice to enable them to manage their bladder problems successfully.

Investigations

Further bladder assessment is sometimes required and this is usually carried out by the continence advisor, uroneurologist or urologist.

Urodynamic investigations may be carried out to try to ascertain what abnormality of function is causing the bladder symptoms. It enables the functions of the bladder, storage and voiding, to be studied.

Uroflowmetry with post void residual

This is measurement of flow rate with ultrasound measurement of the residual urine.

Cystometry

This is measurement of bladder pressure during bladder filling and voiding. Studies have shown that bladder overactivity is the most usual abnormality found in patients with PD. Pressure flow studies are important if obstructive voiding due to an enlarged prostate is suspected (Sakakibara et al 2001).

Sphincter electromyography (EMG)

This is a way of investigating innervation of the pelvic floor. It can be a valuable investigation in the diagnosis of multiple system atrophy (MSA), but it is not widely available in all centres.

Medical management of bladder dysfunction

If the post void residual is less than 100 ml then first line medical management for overactive bladder (urinary frequency and urgency) is usually an oral anticholinergic such as oxybutynin, tolterodine or propantheline. These drugs diminish the parasympathetic innervation of the smooth muscle of the bladder, thereby reducing frequency and urgency. Unfortunately a common side effect is a dry mouth which may be made worse by some antiparkinsonian medication. Those anticholinergics which cross the blood–brain barrier can contribute to confusion and hallucinations so may not be suitable for elderly PD patients or those with existing cognitive impairment. If the patient's residual is more than 100 ml, intermittent self-catheterization may also need to be considered (see Practical management, below).

For many patients nocturnal frequency is a troublesome symptom and cautious use of desmopressin can be useful as it reduces urine production. However, it is contraindicated for use in the elderly.

Urological surgical intervention is generally not indicated in patients with a diagnosis of MSA. Patients with PD who have been shown to have significant prostatic obstruction, however, may benefit from a transurethral resection of the prostate. Patients usually benefit from continuing their anticholinergic medication if they have ongoing symptoms of overactive bladder (Chandiramani and Fowler 1999).

Practical management

The role of the continence advisor

In most areas of the UK there are now nurses or physiotherapists who specialize in continence management. They are available to assess and treat all aspects of bladder and bowel continence. Most continence advisors offer an open referral system that can be accessed by health professionals, patients and their carers. Although they offer a comprehensive service it is always useful for nurses to be aware of the continence strategies available. There are now courses available for nurses for enhancing their practice in this extremely important aspect of patient care.

It is in practical management that the nurse can offer the most effective support for patients and their carers. Knowledge of what is available and how best to apply it to the individual patient can make a significant contribution to the patient's quality of life.

Bladder retraining

Many patients will state that they go to the toilet 'just in case'. If so, it is important to establish a baseline by using a continence chart. Specific charts can be of use to show episodes of urinary frequency and incontinence. The patient and nurse will be more aware of the patient's toileting habit. This can be also used for ongoing assessment of planned management.

Pelvic floor exercises

Most research studies that have been carried out are related to functional problems, such as genuine stress incontinence, other than those caused by neurological dysfunction. It is not known how effective these exercises are in the long term for patients with parkinsonism.

Intermittent self-catheterization

Intermittent self-catheterization (ISC) is the periodic insertion of a non-retaining urinary catheter to empty the bladder. ISC is useful if the patient has incomplete bladder emptying, i.e. a residual urine of over 100 ml. Patients are taught, usually by the continence advisor, to insert the catheter by themselves. Some patients may be unable to do this for themselves, due to tremor, poor eyesight, cognitive impairment or general immobility. In these cases many carers may choose to do it for them. In some areas the district nurses may offer assistance and support for this at home.

The main advantages of ISC are:

- Patient independence
- Risks of indwelling catheter are avoided
- Reduced risk of renal impairment
- Improved bladder symptoms

Some patients may have some initial discomfort and some may develop a urinary tract infection, but, with good aftercare and support, difficulties can be overcome. When considering ISC for a patient, teaching and follow-up are extremely important. Factors to consider when deciding if a patient is suitable for ISC include dexterity, mobility, cognitive function and motivation.

Indwelling or suprapubic catheters

As the disease advances some patients may choose to have an indwelling catheter. Ongoing bladder problems can have a devastating effect on a patient's lifestyle and care, and the introduction of an indwelling catheter can, at times, greatly improve matters. Patients are usually advised to have a suprapubic catheter for long-term management.

The advantages of a suprapubic catheter include:

- No risk of urethral trauma, or related problems
- Greater comfort for PD patients who are chairbound
- Access for cleaning and catheter changing is improved, especially for women
- Catheter-free during sexual activity

The disadvantages of a suprapubic catheter include:

- Surgical procedure
- Patient may have urethral leakage
- Small abdominal incision

An experienced, qualified person should discuss advantages and disadvantages with the patient and carer in advance. The initial suprapubic catheterization is usually carried out under general anaesthetic as a day procedure.

Appliances

Many patients may not wish to perform ISC or have an indwelling catheter. They may be able to contain their incontinence and maintain their quality of life with the help of a continence appliance. There are many different types available and it is important that the patient is offered individual assessment. Advice from a continence advisor and/or a representative of an appliance manufacturing company is extremely important. A useful directory for nurses to have access to is the Continence Foundation's Directory of Continence Products (see Useful addresses).

Absorbent pads and pants
It is important to consider the patient's lifestyle, amount of urine leakage and dependence when choosing a pad. Careful teaching of patients and carers can improve chances of compliant usage of pads and pants. These are available in many sizes and materials, both disposable and reusable.

Urinary sheaths
Some men may choose to have an external drainage system to manage their incontinence, although this does not drain their residual urine. There are many different types of sheath, varying in size and material, and it may take some time to find the most suitable. For patients with a retracted penis, pubic pressure devices with external sheaths are available. A fitting service is available from some manufacturers.

Appliances for women
There is very little available for women apart from catheters and pads. External pouches have been developed but many women find these cumbersome and they can be difficult to apply without considerable instruction and help.

Lifestyle

There are several points concerning lifestyle which should be considered:

- A healthy, well-balanced diet and adequate fluid intake are needed; 1.5–2 litres (6–8 cups per day) should be encouraged. Many patients reduce their fluid intake in the hope of reducing their incontinence. However, concentrated urine can have an irritative effect on the bladder. Also, reduced fluid intake can exacerbate constipation

- Diet and fluid intake may be influenced by patients' ability to swallow and feed themselves
- Clothing could be adapted for ease of access to the toilet. There are many companies that supply suitable clothing and offer ideas for adaptation
- Management of these problems is at times multidisciplinary. Assistance from the dietician, occupational therapist and physiotherapist is often very helpful.

Bowel function

Constipation is reported by 29–67% of patients with PD and difficulty in stool expulsion is reported by 57–67% (Edwards et al 1991; Sakakibara et al 2003). Constipation can be defined as a decrease in frequency of bowel movements to less than three movements a week. The stool may be hard and pellet-like or large and difficult to pass. Constipation and/or faecal incontinence can be a factor in the lives of many otherwise healthy people but it can be an additional problem in the day-to-day management of PD. Not only can constipation affect the patients' general well-being, it can also affect levodopa absorption which, in turn, can exacerbate parkinsonian symptoms (Stocchi 1999; Sakakibara et al 2003).

What goes wrong in Parkinson's disease?

Constipation in PD is probably multifactorial. Stocchi (1999) suggests that it could be due to any or all of the following:

- Functional obstruction due to increased segmental contractions
- Poor colonic contractions (colonic inertia or pseudo-obstruction)
- Functional outlet obstruction
- Weak abdominal staining
- Paradoxical sphincter contraction on defecation resulting in incomplete defecation

In addition to these, there are other factors that may contribute, such as reduced mobility, medication (e.g. anticholinergics), problems with diet or swallowing and general neurological disability (Sakakibara et al 2003).

Some patients additionally experience faecal incontinence. Stocchi (1999) suggests that this maybe caused by the reduced anal tone during resting contraction and voluntary contractions. The inadequate voluntary anal contraction found in PD patients could result in inability to recruit the external anal sphincter muscles.

Assessment of bowel function

It is important that a full assessment is carried out to ascertain the cause of the problem before initiating the correct management. The nurse should consider the following factors when assessing bowel function in patients with PD (reproduced and adapted from Norton and Henry 1999):

- Usual bowel pattern
- Usual stool consistency
- Ability to sense bowel fullness
- Pain before or with defecation
- Urgency and the ability to defer defecation
- Evacuation difficulties: straining, sense of incomplete emptying, digital stimulation or evacuation of stool, use of evacuants
- Passive soiling (loss of stool without a prior urge to defecate)
- Ability to control flatus and distinguish flatus from stool
- Obstetric history
- Bladder control
- Use of pads
- Ability to use the toilet independently
- Toilet adaptations
- Attitude and availability of caregivers
- Effect on lifestyle and relationships
- Psychological factors
- Diet, fluid, swallowing

All the above may have a bearing on how management strategies are instigated.

Investigations and examinations

Not all patients need to undergo the following investigations, but if general management does not result in satisfactory bowel control it may be advisable to find out whether there is a pathophysiological cause of the bowel problem, be it neurogenic or not. Norton and Henry (2001) suggest that all patients with 'disordered defecation' should undergo a sigmoidoscopy no matter what is thought to be the underlying cause. Basic assessment may include:

- Rectal examination. It may be necessary to carry out a digital rectal examination to see if there is faeces in the lower rectum; this also gives gives an indication to the consistency of the stool. It is advisable to read *Digital rectal examination and removal of faeces – Guidance for Nurses* (RCN, 2000).

- Abdominal palpation. Distension and discomfort can be an indication of excess gas, fluid or obstruction

If further investigation is required this may involve anorectal physiology tests and radiology tests.

Management of bowel dysfunction

Accurate diagnosis of the cause of bowel dysfunction is important if the treatment is to be successful in the long term.

Practical management

Before commencing laxatives various factors should be assessed.

Fluid intake
The patient should be encouraged to drink 1.5–2 litres of fluid/day. This will help maintain fluid in the stool, especially if the patient has slow colonic transit. Many people experience a laxative effect when hot drinks are taken.

Diet
A well-balanced diet should be encouraged. This can be difficult to maintain in patients with swallowing difficulties. Lack of fibre is one of the most common reasons for constipation with or without a neurological cause. The input of the dietician is important as an understanding of the types of fibre available within the patient's tolerated diet can have a bearing. A variety of different sources of fibre is helpful in maintaining defecation and general well-being (Edwards 1997).

Position
Good posture while sitting on the toilet is important as it can make passing a motion easier. The patient should sit with the upper body leaning slightly forward, the forearms resting on the thighs, with knees above the hips (the feet may need to be raised off the floor with support).

Facilities and assistance
The use of toilets and facilities should be assessed, both in the hospital and home. Availability of carers, and access to an occupational therapist and physiotherapist for practical and mobility assistance and advice, are helpful for the patient's ongoing management.

Medical management

Individual assessment is essential. If first line nursing management is not effective, medication in the form of laxatives may be necessary. These strategies are not specific to PD patients as no studies have been undertaken to determine regimens in PD. Some commonly used laxatives are listed in Table 7.1.

Table 7.1 Commonly used laxatives

Category	Comments and contraindications	Examples
Bulking agents	Introduce gradually, only after impaction cleared. Avoid if patient has loss of rectal sensation or terminal reservoir syndrome. Ensure sufficient fluid intake	Natural bran Ispaghula husk Methylcellulose Sterculia
Stool softeners	Avoid general use of liquid paraffin	Castor oil Dioctyl sodium sulfo-succinate (osmotic also)
Stimulant/chemical	Use minimal effective dose	Senna Bisacodyl
Osmotic	Flatus may be a problem	Milk of magnesia Lactulose Polyethylene glycol Dioctyl sodium sulfosuccinate (softener also)
Rectally administered aids	Some patients may need assistance or fail to retain	Suppositories (e.g. glycerin, bisacodyl) Enemas (e.g. sodium phosphate-based micro enemas) (Norton and Henry 1999)

The choice of laxative should be determined by the cause of the constipation. For patients with PD who have an inadequate diet, a bulk-forming laxative may be required, together with increased fluid intake. If slow transit is also shown to be a problem, a stimulant could be tried. It is important that all medication is commenced at the minimal dosage as the individual's reaction to laxatives can be varied.

Complementary therapies

Complementary therapies may also have a role to play. These must be discussed with the patient's medical supervisor beforehand. They include (Edwards 1997):

- Colonic massage
- Acupuncture
- Shiatsu
- Herbalism
- Reflexology
- Homeopathy
- Aromatherapy

Further management options

If the use of laxatives, diet and other practical advice are not found to be satisfactory further management options can be considered.

Bowel washouts
Although not routinely carried out in general wards for the management of chronic constipation, these may be effective in some patients. No studies have been carried out in patients with PD.

Manual evacuation
There are some patients for whom this is the only form of evacuation, e.g. patients with spinal cord injury. However, it should only be carried out in specific circumstances (RCN 2000) and by personnel trained to do it.

Surgery
There are various surgical procedures that are available, but no specific data are available in relation to PD patients. A full discussion, by a relevant knowledgeable person, of the perceived benefits and disadvantages needs to take place with the patient and carer before any of these interventions.

Sexual problems

Over the past decade, there have been increasing numbers of reports of sexual problems among neurological patients. These include a small number of studies of patients with PD. Treatment of sexual dysfunction has been revolutionized by the discovery of oral proerectile medication, and the pros and cons of its use in PD patients are starting to be recognized. This should have implications for the previously neglected field of female sexual dysfunction. Nursing input will gradually become better defined, as the psychological, social and medical issues are further highlighted.

Male sexual dysfunction

The prevalence of erectile failure in PD patients has been reported at 60% compared to 37% in age-matched controls in one study (Singer et al 1989). The problem worsens as the disease progresses, and is generally only seen after the diagnosis of PD has been established, unlike MSA in which erectile failure often predates the onset of other neurological symptoms (Beck et al 1994). Other factors, such as psychological influences or prescribed medications, may also be responsible for erectile failure. Conversely, there have also been reports of increased libido following treatment with levodopa or dopamine (DA) agonists (such as apomorphine). Although the cause of erectile failure in PD is not fully elucidated, studies have shown the importance of central dopaminergic (DA-ergic) pathways in penile erection, and the possible pathophysiology of PD involves destruction of DA-containing cells in the substantia nigra; the DA-ergic (D2) agonist apomorphine has been shown to be effective in erectile failure in PD (Stibe et al 1988; O'Sullivan and Hughes 1998).

Treatment

Sildenafil citrate (Viagra®) has been shown to produce erections in patients with PD (Zesiewicz et al 2000). Caution is needed, however, if it is possible that the patient has MSA, since the medication may result in an exacerbation of postural hypotension: these patients are prone to a significant drop in blood pressure when standing from lying down, a symptom that is exacerbated by sildenafil (Hussain et al 2001). The dose prescribed may be 25 mg, 50 mg or 100 mg. Blood pressure (standing and lying) should be measured before commencing treatment.

Sublingual apomorphine (Uprima®) is available for treatment of erectile failure in the general population, at a dose of 3 mg, with a reportedly faster onset of action (within 20 minutes) than sildenafil. However, caution is recommended for patients already on DA-ergic medication, as it is not known whether effects may be potentiated.

Other pharmacological treatments include prostaglandin E1, applied either as an injection (Caverject®) or intra-urethrally (MUSE®). Although these are both efficacious, it should be remembered that they require a degree of manual dexterity, which may limit their practicality.

Ejaculatory delay and difficulty reaching orgasm are also described, and neither is easily overcome.

Female sexual dysfunction

This area has been previously neglected, but general awareness seems to be increasing slowly. The symptoms vary from reduced sexual desire, decreased arousal (i.e. genital lubrication or sensitivity), orgasmic difficulty, to dyspareunia or vaginismus (Basson et al 2000). However, there have been few studies devoted exclusively to female sexuality in PD. Welsh et al (1997) compared 27 women who had PD with age-matched controls, and found the former group to have greater anxiety or inhibition, vaginal tightness, incontinence (with implications for sexual functioning) and dissatisfaction with body appearance; furthermore, the PD patients were less satisfied with their sexual relationship and partners, and more depressed than the control group. However, this study focused on older patients (mean age 67 years). Other issues in sexual function may be relevant for younger patients, such as unemployment or other social factors (Jacobs et al 2000).

Treatments for female sexual dysfunction have been limited generally, and there are no definitive studies in women with PD. Hormonal therapy such as oestrogen (orally or topically) has been used to reduce vaginal dryness and thereby dyspareunia, while testosterone may help increase libido (but is associated with facial hair growth and weight gain). Viagra® has been tried in other female populations with some success (Kaplan et al 1999; Nurnberg et al 1999; Caruso et al 2001), but it is not known whether it will have any benefit for women with PD. As other oral agents are developed for male sexual dysfunction, this may lead to newer therapies for women with the symptoms described.

Nursing contributions

The subject of sexual dysfunction can be initially difficult and embarrassing for both the patient and the health professional. When nursing staff were asked about their views on sexuality counselling, 82% of cardiac nurses felt that sexual counselling after myocardial infarction was within their scope, but did not offer it because they were uncomfortable with this area of education (Shuman and Bohachick 1987). When interviewed, most recipients of sexual counselling felt it was appropriate to be educated by nurses (Waterhouse and Metcalfe 1991). The relationship with a familiar nurse may provide the continuity of care and accessibility that is not always possible within the traditional doctor–patient consultation.

The importance of involving the patient's partner should be highlighted. Brown and co-workers (1990) assessed sexual function in PD patients and their partners in a questionnaire survey; sexual dysfunction was perceived as a problem (by both patient and partner) more frequently when the patient was male. Although the overall level of dissatisfaction in the couples was higher than in the general population, the presence of an identified sexual problem did not always lead to dissatisfaction; this implies that coping strategies were adopted by patient and partner to overcome their difficulty. While depression and anxiety are common in PD patients (Gotham et al 1986), there is also considerable psychological morbidity among those living with and caring for them; this can inevitably lead to additional stress in the sexual relationship. These interpersonal dynamics need time to be explored fully, and involvement of a nurse in a counselling role (or in directing the patient to the appropriate ancillary services) could be considered in the future.

Effective management of bladder, bowel and sexual dysfunction can have a positive influence on the social and psychological aspects of PD. Therefore it is essential that nurses be fully informed if they are to offer complete individualized care. Help is available from many sources and it is important that use is made of these useful resources.

Key points

- Bladder and bowel dysfunction are common in PD and both can have an impact on quality of life
- Bladder symptoms such as urgency and frequency are often worse in the 'off' state
- Nurses should have an understanding of the assessment and management of pelvic organ disorders so that they can offer appropriate care
- Effective management of bladder, bowel and sexual dysfunction can have a positive influence on the social and psychological aspects of PD

Useful addresses

Incontact, United House, North Road, London, N7 9DP.

The Continence Foundation, 307 Hatton Square, 16 Baldwin Gardens, London, EC1N 7RJ.

Promocon/Disabled Living, St Chad Street, Manchester, M8 8QA.

S.P.O.D. (The Association to Aid The Sexual and Personal Relationships of People with a Disability), 286 Camden Road, London, N7 0BJ.

References

Abrams P, Cardozo L, Fall M, Griffiths D, Rosier P, Ulmsten U, van Kerrebroeck P, Victor A and Wein A (2002) The Standardisation of Terminology of Lower Urinary Tract Dysfunction: Report from the Standardisation Sub-committee of the International Continence Society. Neurourology and Urodynamics 21:167–178.

Araki I and Kuno S (2000) Assessment of voiding dysfunction in Parkinson's disease by the international prostate symptom score. Journal of Neurology, Neurosurgery and Psychiatry 68: 429–433.

Basson R, Berman J, Burnett A, Derogatis L, Ferguson D, Fourcroy J, Goldstein I, Graziottin A, Heiman, J, Laan E, Leiblum S, Padma-Nathan H, Rosen R, Segraves K, Segraves R, Shabsigh R, Sipski M, Wagner G and Whipple B (2000) Report of the International Consensus development conference on female sexual dysfunction: definitions and classifications. Journal of Urology 163: 888–893.

Beck R O, Betts C D and Fowler C J (1994) Genito-urinary dysfunction in multiple system atrophy: clinical features and treatment in 62 cases. Journal of Urology 151: 1336–1341.

Brown R, Jahanshahi M, Quinn N and Marsden C D (1990) Sexual function in patients with Parkinson's disease and their partners. Journal of Neurology, Neurosurgery and Psychiatry 53: 480–486.

Caruso S, Intelisano G, Lupo L, Agnello C (2001) Premenopausal women affected by sexual arousal disorder treated with sildenafil: a double-blind, cross-over, placebo-controlled study. British Journal of Obstetrics and Gynaecology 108: 623–628.

Chandiramani V A and Fowler C J (1999) Urogenital disorders in Parkinson's disease and multiple system atrophy. In: C J Fowler (ed.) Neurology of Bladder, Bowel, and Sexual Dysfunction. Boston: Butterworth Heinemann, pp.245–254.

Continence Product Directory, The Continence Foundation, London.

Craggs M D and Vaizey C J (1999) Neurophysiology of the bladder and bowel. In: C J Fowler (ed.) Neurology of Bladder, Bowel and Sexual Dysfunction. Boston: Butterworth Heinemann, pp. 19–32.

Edwards C (1997) Down down and away! An overview of adult constipation and faecal incontinence. In: K Getliff and M Dolman (ed.) Promoting Continence – A Clinical and Research Source. London: Baillière Tindall, pp. 177–226.

Edwards L L, Quigley E, Hofman R and Balluff M (1991) Gastrointerstinal symptoms in Parkinson's disease. Movement Disorders 6(2): 151–156.

Fader M (1997) The promotion and management of continence in neurological disability. In: K Getliff and M Dolman (ed.) Promoting Continence – A Clinical and Research Source. London: Baillière Tindall, pp. 375–409.

Fowler C J (1999) Neurological disorders of micturition and their treatment. Brain 122: 1213–1231.

Gotham A, Brown R and Marsden C D (1986) Depression in Parkinson's disease: a quantitative and qualitative analysis. Journal of Neurology, Neurosurgery and Psychiatry 49: 381–389.

Grimby A, Milsom I, Molander U, Wiklund I and Ekelund P (1993) The influence of urinary incontinence on the quality of life of elderly women. Age and Aging 22: 82–89.

Hussain I F, Brady C M, Swinn M J, Mathias C J and Fowler C J (2001) Treatment of erectile dysfunction with sildenafil citrate (Viagra) in parkinsonism due to Parkinson's disease or multiple system atrophy with observations on orthostatic hypotension. Journal of Neurology, Neurosurgery and Psychiatry 71(3): 371–374.

Jacobs H, Vieregge A and Vieregge P (2000) Sexuality in young patients with Parkinson's disease: a population based comparison with healthy controls. Journal of Neurology, Neurosurgery and Psychiatry 69: 550–552.

Kaplan S A, Reis R B, Kohn I J, Ikeguchi E F, Laor E, Te A E and Martins A C (1999) Safety and efficacy of sildenafil in postmenopausal women with sexual dysfunction. Urology 53(3): 481–486.

Lees A J, Blackburn N A and Campbell V L (1988) The night-time problems of Parkinson's disease. Clinical Pharmacology 11(6): 512–519.

Lubrowski D Z, Swash M and Henry M (1988) Neural mechanisms in disorders of defecation. Baillière's Clinical Gastroenterology 2: 210–223.

Norton C and Henry M (1999) Investigation and treatment of bowel problems. In: C J Fowler (ed.) Neurology of Bladder, Bowel and Sexual Dysfunction. Boston: Butterworth Heinemann, pp. 185–207.

Nurnberg H G, Lauriello J et al (1999) Sildenafil for sexual dysfunction in women taking antidepressants. American Journal of Psychiatry 156(10): 1664.

O'Sullivan J and Hughes A (1998) Apomorphine-induced penile erections in Parkinson's disease. Movement Disorders 3: 536–539.

Raudino F (2001) Non-motor off in Parkinson's disease. Acta Neurologica Scandinavica. 104: 312–315.

Royal College of Nursing (2000) Digital rectal examination and manual removal of faeces – Guidance for nurses.

Sakakibara R, Shinotoh H, Uchiyama T, Sakuma M, Kashiwado M, Yoshiyama M and Hattori T (2001) SPECT imaging of the dopamine transporter with [123 I]-β-CIT reveals marked decline of nigrostiatal dopaminergic function in Parkinson's disease with urinary dysfunction. Journal of Neurological Sciences 187: 55–59.

Sakakibara R, Odaka T, Uchiyama T, Asahina M, Yamaguchi K, Yamaguchi T, Yamanishi T and Hattori T (2003) Colonic transit time and rectoanal videomanometry in Parkinson's disease. Journal of Neurology, Neurosurgery and Psychiatry 74: 268–272.

Shuman N and Bohachick P (1987) Nurses' attitudes towards sexual counselling. Dimensions in Critical Care Nursing 6: 75–81.

Singer C, Weiner W, Sanchez-Ramos J R and Ackerman M (1989) Sexual dysfunction in men with Parkinson's disease. Journal of Neurologic Rehabilitation 3: 199–204.

Stibe C, Kempster P, Lees A J and Stern G M (1988) Subcutaneous apomorphine in parkinsonian on-off fluctuations. Lancet 1(8582): 403–406.

Stocchi F (1999) Disorders of bowel function in Parkinson's disease. In: C J Fowler (ed.) Neurology of Bladder, Bowel, and Sexual Dysfunction. Boston: Butterworth Heinemann, pp. 255–264.

Stocchi F, Badiali D, Vacca L. D,Alba L, Bracci F. Ruggieri S, Torti M, Berardlli A and Corazziari E (2000) Anorectal function in multiple system atrophy and Parkinson's disease. Movement Disorders 15(1): 71–76.

Waterhouse J and Metcalfe M (1991) Attitudes toward nurses discussing sexual concerns with patients. Journal of Advanced Nursing 16: 1048–1054.

Welsh M, Hung L and Waters CH (1997) Sexuality in women with Parkinson's disease. Movement Disorders 12(6): 923–927.

Zesiewicz T A, Helal M, et al (2000). Sildenafil citrate (Viagra) for the treatment of erectile dysfunction in men with Parkinson's disease. Movement Disorders 15(2): 305–308.

CHAPTER EIGHT
Sleep and Parkinson's disease

ELLIE BORRELL

Introduction

Problems with sleep are common in Parkinson's disease (PD) but they are often under-recognized and not adequately assessed or managed. The nursing assessment of PD often tends to focus on daytime problems and how symptoms such as tremor, rigidity and bradykinesia impact on the patient's ability to manage self-care activities. However, sleep is an essential component for healthy living and lack of sleep can significantly affect quality of life. It is only by paying attention to such details as sleep patterns and nocturnal disturbances that one is able to gather an overall picture of a person's quality of life.

This chapter will review normal sleep and the aetiology of sleep disorders and will discuss the specific sleep disorders that can occur in PD. It will also cover the nursing assessment of sleep disorders and provide practical advice on how to promote sleep.

Overview of normal sleep

Only animals with highly developed brains experience sleep. Less developed brains are constantly responding to stimuli so they never fully engage in sleep (Kryger et al 1994). Brain activity continues during sleep but electroencephalograms (EEGs) demonstrate that it differs from that of the waking brain. When we sleep energy is conserved as both metabolism and body temperature decreases. It is thought that this is one of the key factors in mammalian survival (Karni et al 1994). Furthermore, evolution has adapted humans and animals so that we sleep when we will reap the most benefits; temporal and thermal specializations have evolved for survival. It is generally accepted that the main function of sleep is for brain rest but the neurobiology of sleep is still poorly understood.

Sleep/wake cycle

People have professional and social schedules to adhere to and external 'zeitgebers' or time-givers, such as clocks, influence their sleep/wake cycle or 'circadian rhythm'. People adapt their circadian rhythms to suit their lifestyles. However, we also have an additional internal clock which influences our sleep/wake cycle and this is not, as once thought, purely responsive to exogenous stimuli. In the absence of zeitgebers, our bodies continue to run over a period of almost 24 hours, with a cycle of rest and activity and sleep and wake.

The hypothalamus and the brainstem are largely responsible for controlling the sleep/wake cycle. The suprachiasmatic nucleus (SCN) or 'biological clock' is a tiny nucleus located within the hypothalamus (Pickard and Turek 1983). The SCN receives input from the retina and synchronizes circadian rhythms with the daily light–dark cycle.

It is thought that diffuse modulatory neurotransmitter systems are most responsible for the control of sleeping and waking. This means that the neurotransmitters do not directly evoke postsynaptic potential but modify cellular response. The neurotransmitters noradrenaline and serotonin enhance waking, whereas acetylcholine is thought to be particularly critical during rapid eye movement (REM) sleep.

Types of sleep

During normal sleep the brain becomes more active every 90–100 minutes and can remain so for up to an hour. This is the period in which people dream and is called REM sleep. While people sleep, the brain goes through a pattern of REM and non-REM sleep. The hypothalamus and the brainstem are thought to control REM and non-REM sleep.

Non-REM sleep

It is thought that the purpose of non-REM sleep is to rest (Hobson 1995). Muscles are relaxed and movement is infrequent. The brain is able to command movement but only does so occasionally to alter position. The parasympathetic section of the autonomic nervous system increases in activity, and heart rate, respiration and renal function all slow down. The brain is also at rest and it is thought that most sensory input does not even reach the cortex. Dreaming rarely occurs during this phase.

REM sleep

REM sleep is so called because all the muscles in the body are immobilized apart from the eyelids. During REM sleep the brain 'wakes up' and is in an excitable state. This is when people have their most vivid and intricate dreams. During REM sleep the body's core temperature decreases, heart rate and respiration increases and becomes irregular, and the penis and clitoris experience a rush of blood and become erect, but this does not usually indicate dreams of a sexual nature. Overall, to an onlooker the body gives the impression of being asleep when in fact the brain is very active.

Non-REM sleep is seen as a period of rest and energy conservation but the purpose of REM sleep appears to be more complex. Brain activity can be at its height during REM sleep, even more so than when people are awake; clearly the brain is not in a state of rest. The purpose of REM sleep remains poorly understood but it is thought that REM sleep is entirely necessary for a good night's sleep as people who are deprived of REM sleep feel tired and run down.

The aetiology of sleep disorders in PD

Sleep disorders can arise from a variety of mechanisms. For example, the sleep cycle can become unbalanced and this can produce too much, too little or the wrong kind of sleep (Ueyama 1999). Over- or underactivity of the neurones within the SCN nucleus is also thought to be implicated in the aetiology of sleep disorders. It is difficult to pinpoint the exact causes of sleep disorders in PD (Nausieda et al 1982) but it is generally accepted that the main culprits are:

- The disease process
- Dopaminergic (DA-ergic) drugs
- The ageing process

The disease process

Sleep disorders can suddenly occur at any stage in the disease process but they tend to get worse as the disease progresses (Pal et al 1999). The DA depletion and neuronal loss which occur with PD are implicated in the aetiology of the various sleep disorders. There is growing evidence to suggest that DA has an important role to play in the neurobiology of sleep but its exact role is not yet fully understood (Mignot et al 2002).

DA depletion leads to the emergence of tremor, bradykinesia and rigidity, and these symptoms can have an additional impact on sleep.

DA-ergic drugs

DA-ergic medication can have a dramatic effect on sleep patterns (Kales et al 1971), although the precise physiological mechanism remains unclear. It is well recognized that levodopa can cause sleep disruption (Nausieda et al 1982; Factor et al 1990) and this effect is thought to be dose related. Levodopa administered in high doses can cause sleeplessness or insomnia but these high doses tend to be administered later on in the disease and so other factors such as age and disease process may also be contributing to the sleep disturbances. However, lower doses of levodopa can also cause some people to feel excessively sleepy and patients will often complain of this, especially when they first start to take medication.

DA-ergic drugs are also implicated in the aetiology of spontaneous 'sleep attacks' (Frucht et al 1999) but the exact mechanism by which they do so remains poorly understood. Again, it appears to be dose-related.

The ageing process

Sleep disorders tend to be more common in elderly people and this fact is mirrored in PD (Partinen 1997). Sleep patterns change with age and, as we grow older, we generally need less sleep (Williams et al 1974). Elderly people tend to go to sleep earlier and wake up earlier and they will probably experience several periods of wakefulness of varying lengths throughout the night (Pal et al 1999). Furthermore, periodic limb movements, pain and respiratory problems can all affect sleep and these problems tend to become more common with age (Bliwise 1993). Overall, sleep becomes lighter and shorter with age.

However, sleep problems are more common in people with PD than in age-matched controls (Kumar et al 2002) and specific differences are found (Clarenbach 2000). For example, patients with PD generally experience less sleep, poorer quality sleep, an increased number of arousals, more periodic limb movements and sleep-related breathing problems (Mouret 1975). REM behaviour disorder is also more common in the PD population and this may account for the increased incidence of excessive daytime sleepiness (Comella et al 1998).

It is impossible to know if the sleep problems encountered by people with PD are a direct result of the ageing process, but it is more likely that sleep disorders arise from a combination of factors including DA-ergic medication, the disease process and age-related changes.

Sleep problems in PD

Sleep disorders are very common as it is estimated that up to 90% of people with PD can experience sleep problems at some stage of their disease (Happe et al 2001). Sleep disorders can have a profound negative effect on quality of life, from increased anxiety and depression to exacerbation of symptoms (Menza and Rosen 1995). The following sleep disorders will be discussed:

- Insomnia
- Restless legs syndrome
- Periodic leg movements
- REM behaviour disorder
- Excessive daytime sleepiness
- Sleep attacks
- Vivid dreaming and nightmares

Insomnia

A variety of factors is thought to cause insomnia in PD but the main culprits include parkinsonian motor symptoms, nocturia and depression.

Patients often experience a re-emergence of their parkinsonian motor symptoms (tremor stiffness and rigidity) at night, as a result of the wearing-off of their bedtime DA-ergic medication. Symptoms such as rigidity and bradykinesia can cause night-time discomfort and difficulty in turning over, and this can lead to several episodes of wakefulness throughout the night. Furthermore, night-time rigidity often leads to early morning dystonia which can also result in fragmented sleep (Stocchi et al 1998).

Nocturia is also a common reason for sleep disturbance. Lees and others (1988) found that nocturia was the most common cause for sleep disruption in patients with PD. In this study, one third of the patients reported that they had to get up three or more times to pass urine and the remaining two thirds had to get up twice on average during the night. Many patients with PD have reduced or poor mobility at night and this can result in the person suffering from urinary incontinence. This can be very disturbing for patients and their partners.

Depression can occur in up to 40% of people with PD (Tandberg et al 1997) and one strong indication of depression is early morning insomnia (Caap-Ahlgren and Dehlin 2001). Depression is commonly overlooked as PD-associated problems, like sleep disturbance, tend to be linked to more typical PD signs like tremor, rigidity and bradykinesia (Menza and Rosen 1995). There are two main causes of depression in PD. The first is a reactive depression, which is linked to a person's reaction to their diagnosis and the impact their disease has on their activities of daily living (Caap-Ahlgren and Dehlin 2001). It is quite normal for someone to feel depressed when they receive a diagnosis of PD (Allain et al 2000). The role of the Parkinson's disease Nurse Specialist (PDNS) in this situation is invaluable. Secondly, the neurochemical changes which occur in PD can also result in depression, especially in the later stages of disease (Choi et al 2000). Antidepressants are often prescribed to good effect, the most favoured being selective serotonin re-uptake inhibitors (SSRIs) (Hauser et al 1997). Amitriptyline is also sometimes prescribed as it is used in depressive illness and also has a sedative effect.

Restless legs syndrome (RLS)

RLS is a common nocturnal complaint which can also occur in people who do not have PD (Lang 1987). RLS typically occurs late in the evening or during the night and is described as a sensation like pins and needles which forces a person to get up and walk about to relieve the discomfort. This can be made worse by night-time rigidity, making it difficult or impossible for a person to mobilize and therefore obtain relief. The aetiology of RLS remains unclear but patients often report positive results with levodopa treatment (Akpinar 1982). Over time, however, people experience a worsening of symptoms, with the condition being particularly severe before the evening dose of levodopa (Lang 1987).

RLS typically occurs in people with PD who are over 65 years of age (Comella 2002) but one study exploring RLS in the general population found the mean age of onset was 27 years (Montplaisier et al 1997). RLS can occur at any stage in the disease but it has been known to precede other parkinsonian symptoms by a number of years (Lang 1987). RLS tends to be similar to PD, as it is a long-term condition which worsens with age (Factor et al 1990).

Periodic leg movements

Another similar nocturnal complaint, but less common, is periodic leg movements. The person experiences violent movements of their arms and legs during REM sleep and this can result in injury.

REM behaviour disorder (RBD)

RBD is characterized by excessive motor activity during the dreaming phase of sleep. It is associated with loss of skeletal muscle atonia in REM sleep (Olson et al 2000). Patients can experience vivid dreams which they act out, and symptoms can include punching, shouting and, in some cases, attempted strangulation of the spouse (Tan et al 1996). Often partners will report violent physical outbursts during sleep and it is not uncommon for them to receive a black eye as a result. Couples may end up sleeping in separate beds and this can obviously have a significant effect on their quality of life.

Periodic leg movements are also seen to be a feature of RBD, but RBD presentation and diagnosis is not limited to merely limb movement. Although RBD can be found in several areas of the population, most typically in elderly men, it is also strongly associated with PD (Schenck et al 1996). RBD can be successfully treated with clonazepam and it is worth considering treatment in those patients who put themselves or others at risk.

Excessive daytime sleepiness (EDS)

EDS is another common and equally troublesome problem associated with PD (Reyner and Horne 1998). People who experience EDS generally complain of severe tiredness and fatigue and it is not unusual for people to sleep for up to 2 or 3 hours both in the morning and in the afternoon. Obviously this can have an enormous consequence for the patients as it can affect their lifestyle and relationships.

EDS can be caused by insomnia, poor quality night-time sleep and DA-ergic medication. Although levodopa improves sleep by easing parkinsonian motor symptoms, insomnia and somnolence are known side effects (Lees et al 1989). Patients often complain of EDS, particularly on lower doses of levodopa, and this is thought to be due to the alteration of serotonergic and DA-ergic mechanisms induced by levodopa therapy (Happe et al 2001). Paradoxically, patients on higher doses of levodopa can also experience problems with insomnia (Nausieda et al 1982).

Sleep attacks

A relatively recently reported phenomenon is that of 'sleep attacks' (falling asleep without warning). Sleep attacks were initially thought to be caused by the newer DA agonists such as pramipexole and ropinirole (Moller et al 2002) but it is now generally accepted that all DA-ergic drugs, including levodopa, can potentially cause this problem. Sleep attacks are potentially very serious as there have been reports of people falling asleep while driving, and causing accidents (Frucht et al 1999). Patients should therefore be given comprehensive advice about the possible problems associated with their medication, particularly agonists, and be advised not to drive if sleep attacks they experience.

Vivid dreaming and nightmares

Patients with PD or, more notably, their partners, often complain of nightmares. Vivid dreaming and nightmares occur most often in patients who have had PD for several years and who have been on levodopa or other DA-ergic medication for some time (Partinen 1997). It is important to take note if a patient reports nightmares, as this could be a precursor to other drug-related problems, such as hallucinations, psychosis or PD-associated conditions, such as Lewy body dementia (Arnulf et al 2000).

Nursing assessment of sleep

Sleep deprivation and excessive sleepiness can have a dramatic effect on quality of life for both patients and their partners. Not surprisingly, sleep problems in partners are as common as in patients (Smith et al 1997).

In order to provide the most effective intervention, it is important to understand the exact nature of the problem and how it affects both the patient's and the partner's quality of life. Four hours' sleep to one person may be perfectly acceptable whereas another could consider it as insomnia. Once a sleep problem is recognized then the nurse can work with the patient to identify a possible cause. The questions listed in Table 8.1 might help identify sleep problems and their possible causes.

Table 8.1 Suggested questions to identify sleep problems

- What is the patient's usual bedtime routine?
- What time does the patient go to bed and get up?
- How often does the patient wake up during the night and for how long?
- Is the patient experiencing violent nightmares?
- Has the patient's partner noticed anything unusual about the patient's pattern of sleep?
- Does the patient take any coffee, tea or alcohol before going to bed?
- How often does the patient have to get up at night to pass urine?
- Does the patient experience any daytime somnolence?
- How long has the patient experienced problems with sleep?
- How often does the sleep disruption occur?
- Is the carer's sleep affected?
- How is the patient's mood?

The Epworth Sleepiness Scale (Johns 1991) is a useful tool which can enable the clinician or nurse to establish the degree of sleep deprivation and EDS. A score of more than 16 is considered to be indicative of a serious problem.

Treatment of sleep problems

For some, the obvious treatment of insomnia is to prescribe sedatives, but these drugs are not without their problems and so are usually only helpful on a short-term basis and should be avoided as far as possible.

To treat a sleep problem accurately one must identify the cause, e.g. bladder symptoms, nocturnal stiffness or rigidity, or depression. If any these are identified then they should be properly assessed and managed in turn. The patient's medication regimen should also be examined. Often by advising a patient not to take levodopa after 7pm, for example, one can help alleviate or at least improve problems associated with vivid dreams and nightmares. However, this can create problems with night-time rigidity, so the physician and the PD nurse, together with the patient, should carefully discuss the advantages and the disadvantages of the various approaches.

If the patient is experiencing EDS, it must be established whether the patient is excessively sleepy during the day because of drug therapy or because of inability to sleep at night. Establishing the cause and the effect is essential before treatment and advice can be offered.

The nurse is in an ideal position to offer patients and their partners practical advice on promoting sleep and simple advice is shown in Table 8.2.

Table 8.2 Practical advice to promote sleep

- Avoid stimulants such as caffeine and alcohol before bedtime
- Try not to eat a large meal immediately before going to bed
- Adopt a bedtime routine and try to go to bed at the same time every night
- If you experience EDS, try an afternoon nap for a planned time – PD often responds well to this
- Relaxation and yoga can help prepare you for sleep
- Take regular exercise

Conclusion

There are many different causes of sleep disorders in PD and many different ways in which they can manifest. Comprehensive knowledge of normal sleep and the various sleep disorders that can occur in PD is useful in providing an informed and holistic assessment. A full and detailed assessment by the nurse can help the patient tackle the problem areas and thus enable the patient and partner to enjoy an improved quality of life and a good night's sleep.

Key points

- It is estimated that up to 90% of people with PD experience sleep problems at some stage of their disease
- Sleep disorders in PD are thought to be caused by a combination of factors including the ageing process, the disease process and DA-ergic medication

- Patients with PD can experience a variety of sleep disorders: insomnia, excessive daytime sleepiness, sleep attacks and vivid dreaming and nightmares
- Sleep deprivation and excessive sleepiness can have a dramatic effect on quality of life for both patients and their partners
- A full and detailed assessment by the nurse can help identify problem areas

References

Akpinar S (1982) Treatment of restless legs syndrome with levodopa plus benzerazide. Archives of Neurology 39:739.

Allain H, Schuck S and Maudit N (2000) Depression in Parkinson's disease. British Medical Journal 320(7245): 1287–1288.

Arnulf I, Bonnet A M, Damier P, Bejjani B P, Seilhean D, Derenne J P and Agid Y (2000) Hallucinations, REM sleep, and Parkinson's disease. Neurology 55(2): 281–288.

Bliwise D L (1993) Sleep in normal aging and dementia. Sleep 16: 40–81.

Caap-Ahlgren M and Dehlin O (2001) Insomnia and depressive symptoms in patients with Parkinson's disease. Relationship to health related quality of life. An interview study of patients living at home. Archives of Gerontology and Geriatrics 32(1): 23–33.

Choi C, Sohn Y, Lee J and Kim J (2000) The effect of long-term therapy on depression level in de novo patients with Parkinson's disease. Journal of the Neurological Sciences 172(1): 12–16.

Clarenbach P (2000) Parkinson's disease and sleep. Journal of Neurology 247(Suppl 4): 20–23.

Comella C L (2002) Restless legs syndrome: treatment with dopaminergic agents. Neurology 58(4 Suppl 1): S87–92.

Comella C L, Nardine T M, Diederich M J and Stebbins G T (1998) Sleep related violence, injury, and REM sleep behaviour disorder in Parkinson's disease. Neurology 51: 526–529.

Factor S A, McAlarney T, Sanchez-Ramos J R and Weiner W J (1990) Sleep disorders and sleep effects in Parkinson's Disease. Movement Disorders 5(4): 280–285.

Frucht S, Rogers J D, Greene P E, Gordon M F and Fahn S (1999) Falling asleep at the wheel: motor vehicle mishaps in persons taking pramipexole and ropinirole. Neurology 52: 1908–1910.

Happe S, Shrodi B, Faltl M, Muller C, Auff E and Zeitlhofer J (2001) Sleep disorders and depression in patients with Parkinson's disease. Acta Neurologica Scandinavica 104: 275–280.

Hauser R A and Zesiewicz T A. (1997) Sertraline for the treatment of depression in Parkinson's disease. Movement Disorders 12(5): 756–759.

van Hilten J J, Weggeman M, van de Velde E A, Kerkhof G A, van Dijk J G and Roos R A C (1993) Sleep, excessive daytime sleepiness and fatigue in Parkinson's disease. Journal of Neural Transmission 5(3): 235–244.

Hobson J A (1995) Sleep. New York: Scientific American Library.

Johns M W (1991) A new method for measuring daytime sleepiness: The Epworth Sleepiness Scale. Sleep 14: 540–545.

Kales A, Ansel R D, Markham C H, Scharf M B and Tan T L (1971) Sleep in patients with Parkinson's disease and normal subjects prior to and following levodopa administration. Clinical Pharmacology and Therapeutics 12(2): 397–406.

Karni A, Tanne D, Rubenstein B S, Askenasy J J M and Sagi D (1994) Dependence on REM sleep of overnight improvement of a perceptual skill. Science 265: 679–682.

Kryger M H, Rot T and Dement W C (1994) The Principles and Practice of Sleep Medicine. Philadelphia: WB Saunders.

Kumar S, Bhatia M and Behari M (2002) Sleep disorders in Parkinson's disease. Movement Disorders 17(4): 775–781.

Lang A E (1987) Restless legs syndrome and Parkinson's disease: insights into pathophysiology. Clinical Neuropharmacology 10(5): 476–478.

Lees A J, Blackburn N A and Campbell V L (1988) The nighttime problems of Parkinson's disease. Clinical Neuropharmacology 11: 512–519.

Menza M and Rosen R (1995) Sleep in Parkinson's disease – the role of depression and anxiety. Psychosomatics 36: 262–266.

Mignot E, Taheri S and Nishino S (2002) Sleeping with the hypothalamus: emerging therapeutic targets for sleep disorders. Nature Neuroscience 5(supp): 1071–1075.

Moller J C, Stiasny K, Hargutt V, Cassel W, Tietze H, Peter J H, Kruger H P and Oertal W H (2002) Evaluation of sleep and driving performance in six patients with Parkinson's disease reporting sudden onset of sleep under dopaminergic medication: a pilot study. Movement Disorders 17(3): 474–481.

Montplaisir J, Boucher S, Poirier G, Lavigne G, Lapierrie O and Lisperance P (1997) Clinical polysomnographic and genetic characteristics of restless legs syndrome: a study of 133 patients diagnosed with new standard criteria. Movement Disorders 12: 61–65.

Mouret J (1975) Differences in sleep in patients with Parkinson's disease. Electroencephalography and Clinical Neurophysiology 38: 653–657.

Nausieda P A, Weiner W J, Kaplan L R, Weber S and Klawans H L (1982) Sleep disruption in the course of chronic L-dopa therapy: an early feature of levodopa psychosis. Clinical Neuropharmacology 5(suppl 2): 183–194.

Olson E J, Boeve B F and Silber M H (2000) Rapid eye movement sleep behaviour disorder: demographic, clinical and laboratory findings in 93 cases. Brain 123(2): 331–339.

Pal S, Bhattacharya K F, Agapito C, Chaudhuri R K (2000) A study of excessive daytime sleepiness and its clinical significance in three groups of Parkinson's disease patients taking pramipexole, cabergoline and levodopa mono and combination therapy. Journal of Neural Transmission 108: 71–77.

Pal P K, Calne S, Samii A and Fleming J A E (1999) A review of normal sleep and its disturbances in Parkinson's disease. Parkinsonism and Related Disorders 5: 1–17.

Partinen M (1997) Sleep disorder related to Parkinson's disease. Journal of Neurology 244(suppl 1): S3–6.

Pickard G E and Turek F K (1983) The suprachiasmatic nuclei: two circadian clocks? Brain Research 268: 201–210.

Reyner W and Horne J (1998) Falling asleep whilst driving: are drivers aware of prior sleepiness? International Journal of Legal Medicine 111: 120–123.

Schenck C H, Bundlie S R and Mahowald M W (1996) Delayed emergence of a parkinsonian disorder in 38% of 29 older men initially diagnosed with idiopathic rapid eye movement sleep behaviour disorder. Neurology 46: 293–393.

Smith M C, Ellgring H and Oertel W H (1997) Sleep disturbances in Parkinson's disease patients and spouses. Journal of American Geriatricians Society 45(2): 194–199.

Stocchi F, Barbato L, Nordera G, Berardelli A and Ruggieri S (1998) Sleep disorders in Parkinson's disease. Journal of Neurology 245(suppl 1): S15–18.

Tan A, Sagad M and Fahn S (1996) Rapid eye movement sleep behaviour disorder preceding Parkinson's disease with therapeutic response to levodopa. Movement Disorders 11(2): 214–216.

Tandberg E, Larson J P, Aarsland D, Laake K and Cummings J L (1997) Risk factors for depression in Parkinson's disease. Archives of Neurology 54: 625–630.

Ueyama T (1999) Suprachiasmatic nucleus: a central autonomic clock. Nature Neuroscience 2: 1051–1053.

Williams R L, Karacan I and Hursch C H (1974) EEG of human sleep. Clinical Applications. New York: Wiley.

CHAPTER NINE

Communication and swallowing in Parkinson's disease

GABRIELLE IRWIN

The purpose of this chapter is to describe how and why people with Parkinson's disease (PD) experience both communication and swallowing disorders, and the clinical signs that warrant speech and language therapy involvement. Included in each section is a brief outline of normal communication and swallowing, followed by current assessment tools and treatment techniques that have been found to be effective in therapy. Consideration of drooling is included.

Introduction

Communication and swallowing disorders in PD occur as a result of the neurological changes that occur within the basal ganglia and which manifest themselves in the features associated with PD: tremor, bradykinesia and rigidity.

Communication and swallowing disorders may be compounded by the effects of medication. In the initial stages of the disease, fluctuations in motor skills are often related to the length of time in which the medication is effective. As the disease progresses, such fluctuations become more severe and are known commonly as the 'on' and 'off' phenomena. In addition, the development of dyskinesias may adversely affect communication and swallowing competence.

Communication

Communication is an inherent part of our identity. It is used to convey our thoughts and ideas, to express our needs, to exchange information, to establish personal contact with others and, often, to demonstrate our capacity to 'fit in' amongst our peers and contemporaries. How we communicate to those around us contributes to how we are perceived as individuals.

The natural rhythm of interaction requires initiation and completion of both voluntary and involuntary motor sequences. Of the features mentioned above, bradykinesia, or slowness of movement, is said to impact the most on human interaction (Klasner and Yorkston 2000). The inability to initiate and perform voluntary movement sequences in response to visual, auditory or tactile stimuli disrupts the natural rhythm of interaction and, as a result, communication breaks down to varying degrees. People with PD frequently find that the spontaneous non-verbal response of a smile or a frown, a shrug of the shoulder or a nod, at best occurs in a slow and deliberate fashion, or at worst is non-existent. Resting tremors, rigidity and the unpredictable involuntary dyskinetic movements further interrupt the continuity of dialogue. Speech may become less 'fluent' and the words less intelligible to the listener. The loss of these communication skills has a profound effect on the quality of life for all concerned. Communication difficulties may thus create a misleading impression of the person with PD who may be seen as being difficult, deaf, drunk or unintelligent (Scott 1998). For the person with PD it is the fundamental loss of control over the motor movements that causes frustration. For the interactive partner, it is the loss of the perceived individual.

Communication requires the simultaneous coming together of different components:

- Speech: the ability to manipulate the vocal tract in order to create sequences of sounds to form words and phrases
- Prosody: the ability to place appropriate intonation, stress and rate on spoken words
- Language: the shared system of coding that manifests itself in the spoken or written word, gesture or symbol. This can be verbal or non-verbal
- Cognition: the ability to concentrate and attend, process perceptual information, intellectually problem solve, use short- and long-term memory and employ self-awareness
- Motivation: the desire to communicate in the environment

In the following section, the impact of PD on each of these components and hence interaction as a whole, is described.

Speech impairments in Parkinson's disease

The type of speech problem associated with PD is *dysarthria*. This is a general term that refers to an entire group of motor speech disorders which result from impaired muscular control of the speech mechanism. The specific type of dysarthria characteristic of PD is called *hypokinetic dysarthria*. It is estimated that 60–80% of people with PD present with this type of dysarthria, with the prevalence increasing as the disease progresses

(Scott et al 1985; Johnson and Pring 1990). Oxtoby (1982) goes on to suggest that over 75% of people with parkinsonism eventually develop speech and voice deficits that decrease their ability to communicate with family and friends, and limit the opportunity for employment.

Characteristics of hypokinetic dysarthria

Marigliani et al (1998) described four groups of 'speech' deficits in PD. Included are the deficits attributed to language and cognition. These are listed below with some of the corresponding features that are frequently observed (adapted from Marks et al 2001a).

Voice

- Reduced respiratory support for volume and phonation
- Harsh, breathy, whispery voice quality
- Limited or reduced ability to signal intonation, resulting in monotonous speech
- Disturbed resonance, often hypernasal

Fluency

- Stuttering-like speech pattern, often termed 'festination'
- Sound, syllable or word repetitions
- Initial word blocks and difficulty in initiating words
- Increased number of pauses
- Listener's perception of rapid speech

Articulation

- Imprecise consonants and vowels resulting in 'slurred' speech

Language and cognition

- Reduced auditory comprehension of sentences and complex commands
- Reduced syntactic complexity in spontaneous speech
- Reduced initiation of conversation
- Inappropriate cessation of sentences
- Disrupted thought planning and sequencing
- Decreased insight and self-monitoring skills
- Reduced ability in topic maintenance
- Impaired memory resulting in difficulties in learning and relearning
- Reduced visuospatial skills

Depression
In addition to the above, research has suggested that up to 47% of people with PD present with depression (Dooneief et al 1992). Depression,

characterized by pessimism and hopelessness, decreased motivation and drive, has implications for social interaction and communication (Klasner and Yorkston 2000).

Writing

In a study by Longstreth et al (1992), 75% of people with PD agreed with the statement 'I am having trouble writing or typing'. The condition of having of small, sometimes, illegible handwriting is known as *micrographia*. This can significantly reduce an individual's ability to use this means of communication either directly, as in correspondence, or as a breakdown resolution strategy when speech becomes unintelligible.

Speech and language therapy intervention

Referral

Timing of intervention is important. Commonly, many people with PD do not seek advice for their speech deficits until they are seen to impact significantly on their ability to communicate. Berry (1983) suggests that referral for therapy should occur prior to the emerging dysarthria, and many therapists advocate a 'sooner rather than later' approach. Cognitive impairment is more likely to occur in advanced disease and this might impact on the patient's ability to learn new skills and generalize these to the home environment.

In a hospital setting, referrals can be made by any member of the multidisciplinary team alerting the medical team to the difficulties an individual is experiencing. Whilst therapy for communication disorders often takes place within a community setting, referrals during a hospital admission are invaluable for establishing the role of the speech and language therapist to the person with PD. Generally, as in the case of most progressive neurological diseases, referral to the community therapist is made after discharge, thus ensuring regular follow-up and support where needed.

Quantity and frequency of intervention

Research has suggested that periods of intensive therapy, between 2 and 4 weeks on a daily or slightly less frequent basis, provide the most effective outcomes (Scott and Caird 1983; Johnson and Pring 1990; Ramig et al 1994). Such intensive programmes are generally then followed up by refresher courses to ensure ongoing motivation, monitoring and maintenance of acquired skills.

Assessment and treatment

Effective treatment of hypokinetic dysarthria is determined by a detailed assessment of the individual's speech mechanism. Formal perceptual assessments commonly used include the Frenchay Dysarthria Assessment (Enderby 1980) or the Assessment of Intelligibility of Dysarthric Speech (Yorkston and Beukleman 1981). Acoustic and physiological measures of assessment are less frequent in general practice for hypokinetic dysarthria. For a detailed description of these, the reader is directed to Murdoch (1998).

The focus and content of treatment programmes will vary with the individual dysarthric profile that is gained from the assessment. All programmes will aim to teach straightforward exercises and strategies that encourage conscious attention to the specific presenting speech pattern observed. Following an explanation of the vocal tract mechanism, exercises for facial expression, breathing and voice, volume, rate of speech, stress, intonation and articulation may all be covered in the programme.

In addition to exercises, compensatory strategies may also be given. Again, these are exclusive to the individual's unique speech pattern. For those who have rapid speech, examples of these might include verbal or written prompts to:

- Speak one word at a time
- Break up the sentence into phrases
- Pause between each word
- Exaggerate the first, middle and/or last letter of each word

Some people with a rapid rate of speech have found that a 'pacing board' assists in breaking up the message into smaller units. A pacing board is, simply, a rectangular block of wood that is divided into five sections. Individuals are asked to point to each section on the pacing board each time they say the initial word of a phrase. This has the effect of slowing down the rate of speech.

Similarly, a metronome can provide an auditory cue to initiate a word. Although the rhythmic pattern of the speech sounds is altered, people with PD have been known to improve intelligibility through this means.

The Lee Silverman Voice Treatment Programme

Recently, people with PD have reported success in generalizing speech improvements from the clinic to the home environment through 'The Lee Silverman Voice Treatment Programme' (Ramig et al 1995). This programme is intensive, and requires the individual to produce a 'loud voice' with 'maximum effort' during speech tasks. Self-monitoring of the level of 'loudness' of the voice and the effort necessary to maintain this are seen as integral aspects of the therapy and, as such, are emphasized and encouraged throughout.

Communication aids

Communication aids to assist intelligibility have been used with varying success with some patients with PD. However, it is a common misconception for many patients that the provision of a communication aid will resolve all their communication problems. It is essential that a specialist speech and language therapist is involved before the purchase or provision of any aid, in order to assess whether the individual has the necessary knowledge, skills and judgement for its use. In addition, it should be remembered that, as PD is progressive, the needs and requirements of an individual will change over time. Hence it is highly unlikely that any one aid will be relevant for the duration of the communication disorder. Often the use of two or three different aids assists the individual as different presentations of the disease occur. Ongoing assessment and re-evaluation of skills, training, support and maintenance are crucial if an individual is to succeed functionally in using aids of any description.

Pen and paper

The use of a pen and paper either to augment or substitute for speech is an appropriate strategy for some people with PD. Whilst conventionally it is associated with full text, the use of a pen and paper in this instance can serve as a shorthand. The individual may chose to write only an initial letter or a key word of the sentence, or draw a representation of the word in picture form.

Alphabet charts

Alphabet charts can be used when a patient is able to point either to the initial letter of a word (to cue the spoken word), or to all of the letters in a word. When an individual is unable to finger point, success may be achieved through eye pointing to the letters. Typed lists of frequently used phrases can also be accessed in the same way.

Electronic communication aids

Electronic communication aids, including dedicated systems (such as a Lightwriter, Figure 9.1) or a portable computer with speech synthesizer, may be useful where a person becomes totally unintelligible but retains the motor ability to use a keyboard. Electronic aids can also be indirectly accessed through a switch that is activated by a single volitional movement (such as an eye blink or finger tap). In the latter case, the individual is required to 'scan' a visual alphabet on the screen of the communication aid.

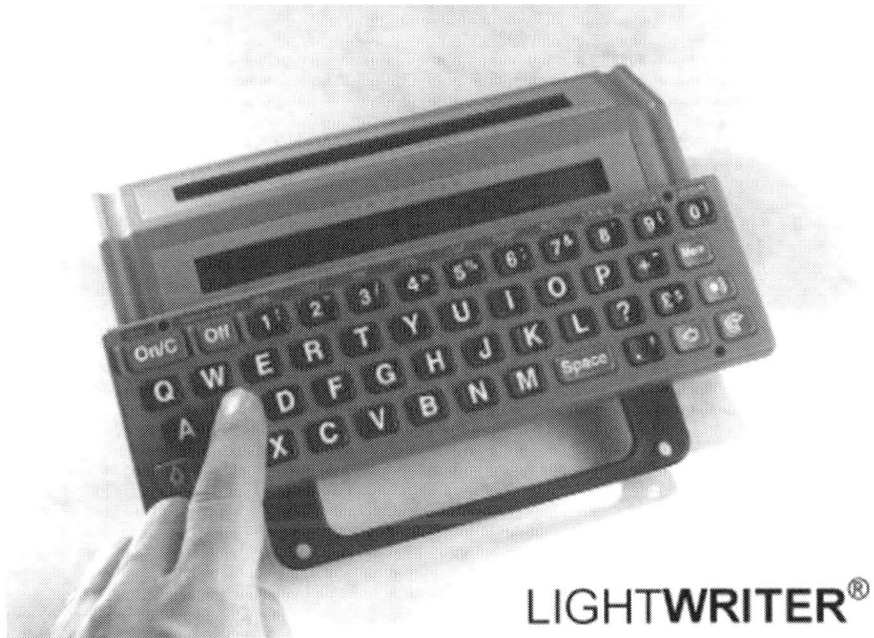

Figure 9.1 Lightwriter SL35 (reproduced with permission of Lightwriter).

Voice amplification aids

Voice amplification aids are useful for patients who experience purely reduced volume of their speech in the absence of slurring. These consist of a small microphone attached to an adjustable arm, which is connected to either a headband or spectacles. This is connected to a low-powered amplifier, which is encased and can be worn on a belt (Figure 9.2).

The environment and interactive nature of communication

It is important to remember that communication always takes place within a context and an environment. An understanding of the nature of the communication disorder by those who interact with the person with PD is essential if appropriate support is to be given. Many people with PD report that some very fundamental and basic strategies are particularly helpful in making their environment conducive to conversation. Some of these are listed in Table 9.1.

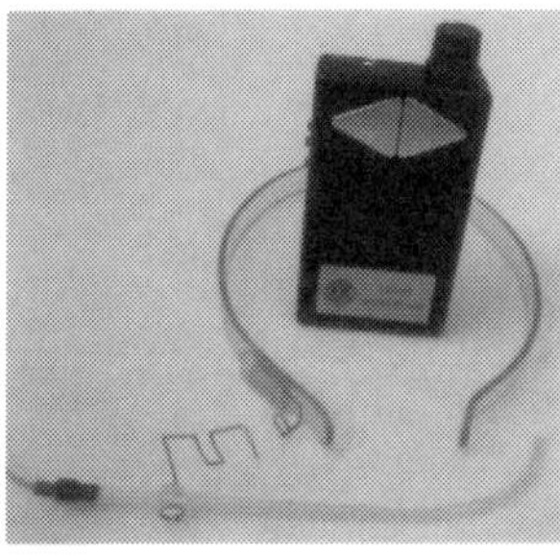

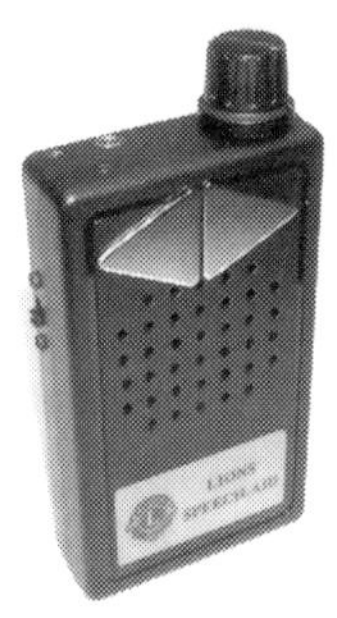

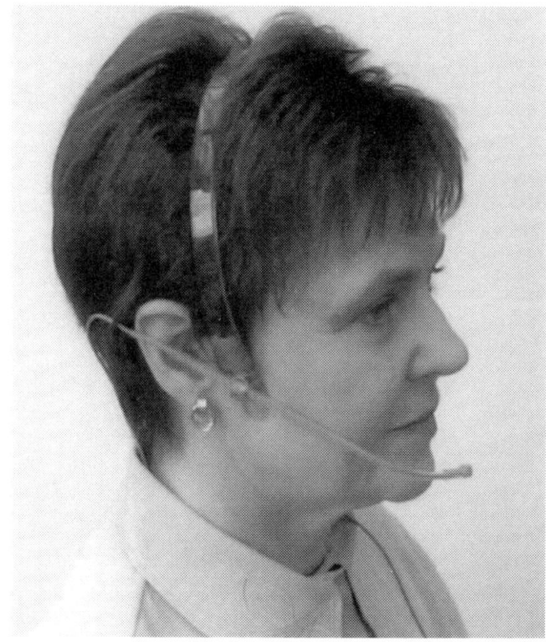

Figure 9.2 Voice amplifier (reproduced with permission by David Lloyd, Lions speech aid).

Table 9.1 Basic strategies that promote an environment conducive to conversation

- Preparing the environment by turning down external distractions such as the television and ensuring good lighting
- Positioning the interactive partner so that, where possible, they are seated opposite and, if culturally appropriate, at the same eye level
- Reducing the number of people who may be speaking and requiring responses from the individual at the same time
- Clarifying what is understood to have been said and acknowledge what has not been understood
- Allowing extra time for the individual to process information
- Allowing extra time for the individual to form their thoughts and speak
- Establishing a consistent verbal or non-verbal 'yes' or 'no' response
- Avoid answering questions on behalf of the person with PD
- Assisting with any of the strategies outlined above, e.g. with syllable pacing or the use of an alphabet chart
- Providing opportunities to communicate rather than making choices for the individual
- Waiting for an appropriate time, perhaps when the person with PD is 'on', to ask questions that require a more detailed response

Swallowing

The normal swallow

The physiology of the normal swallow process is highly complex. It consists, classically, of four phases.

Oral preparatory phase

During this phase a bolus is placed in the mouth and, depending on the taste, consistency and texture, it is moved around the mouth in preparation for mastication to take place. Saliva assists in forming a bolus where necessary. Before initiating the swallow trigger, the food is pulled together to form a semi-cohesive bolus. During this phase, lip seal is usually maintained and the soft palate is lowered against the back of the tongue to maintain bolus position within the oral cavity. Tension in the buccal musculature, or cheeks, prevents food falling into the lateral sulcus between the cheek and mandible.

Oral phase

During the oral phase of the swallow a central groove is formed in the tongue. This acts as a chute for food to pass along as the tongue squeezes the bolus backwards. The buccal musculature tenses slightly to assist this, and lip seal must be maintained. This phase ends as the bolus passes the anterior faucal arches.

Pharyngeal phase

For most people, the pharyngeal phase begins with the triggering of the swallow reflex at the anterior faucal arches. As this occurs, the soft palate rises to close off the nasopharynx from the oral cavity; the larynx elevates and moves forward and closes the airway at three sphincters – the true vocal folds, the false vocal folds and the epiglottis. Finally, the cricopharyngeal sphincter opens in response to the forward and upward motion of the hyoid bone, to allow the bolus entry to the oesophagus.

Oesophageal phase

During this phase, oesophageal peristalsis carries the bolus through the cervical and thoracic oesophagus and into the stomach.

Swallowing impairments in Parkinson's disease

Swallowing difficulties are medically referred to as dysphagia and it is estimated that between 50% and 80% of people with PD suffer from it to

Table 9.2 Signs of dysphagia

- Loss of appetite
- Weight loss
- Fear and anxiety of choking
- Reduced social contact due to embarrassment
- Prolonged mealtimes sometimes requiring assistance
- Packing food into the oral cavity
- Choking at night
- Drooling
- Disturbed intake of medication
- Coughing in the absence of 'chest infection'
- Spiking temperatures
- Bronchopneumonia

different degrees (Leopald and Kagel 1996). Overt signs and symptoms of dysphagia are shown in Table 9.2.

Where end-stage PD results in dementia, individuals may not be able to remember to swallow, nor be able to learn any strategies that may help to prevent choking. Without the 'cognitive drive' to transport the food, it often remains in the mouth for prolonged periods.

Medical implications

The medical implications of dysphagia are that, if it is untreated or inappropriately managed, serious swallowing difficulties can occur. Aspiration pneumonia occurs when food or fluid passes into the laryngeal vestibule, past the vocal folds and into the trachea. This can be detected at the bedside through persistent coughing or choking and/or from changes in the vocal quality, which may sound wet or 'gurgly' after the swallow. If aspiration occurs regularly, the person with PD often experiences spiking temperatures and repeated chest infections. Due to reduced sensation, people with PD are not always aware that dysphagia may be occurring and as a result do not always cough in a reflex response to particles in the larynx or trachea. This is termed silent aspiration.

Common swallowing characteristics

Patients with rigidity, tremor or bradykinesia often experience difficulties in the following aspects of swallowing (adapted from Logemann 1998):

- Maintaining good posture for swallowing because of impaired trunk, head and neck positioning and/or dyskinesias
- Bolus placement because of inability to initiate the required movement, or direct the bolus to the oral cavity as a result of upper limb dismobility

- Preparing the bolus into a compact 'ball', because of reduced lip seal, reduced tongue mobility and jaw rigidity
- Transporting the bolus from the anterior to posterior oral cavity as a result of tongue 'pumping'. This occurs when the back of the tongue does not lower sufficiently for the bolus to pass over its surface. The result is that the bolus is moved forward and back to the middle of the tongue in the oral cavity
- Triggering of the swallow with a timely delay of 2–3 seconds. This can cause the bolus to escape prematurely into the pharynx and then into the open laryngeal vestibule. Coughing *before* the trigger of swallow is then observed
- Obtaining appropriate pressure to force the bolus into the pharynx because of an insufficient seal between the pharyngeal wall and the base of tongue. This may result in residue in the valleculae and pyriform sinuses following each swallow. Residue may accumulate with each successive swallow, and if it is not cleared effectively it can fall into the airway when the individual inhales. This can cause coughing *after* the swallow
- Obtaining elevation and closure of the larynx, as a result of insufficient involvement of the laryngeal musculature. In this instance material can enter the laryngeal vestibule *during* the swallow procedure
- Clearing the bolus from the pharynx and suffering oesophageal reflux due to impairment in either the cricopharyngeal, or upper oesophageal sphincter

Assessment of dysphagia

Case history

It is important for the speech and language therapist to take a detailed case history when investigating any swallowing problems. This will ascertain the length and severity of the problem and provide the foundations from which to treat the dysphagia. Much information can be gained through guided investigation and self-reported difficulties.

Observation

Following the case history, the therapist should observe the individual to assess their eating and drinking. Where possible this should take place in as natural a setting as possible. In a hospital, observation during set mealtimes is not always appropriate, particularly if the patient is on trials of medication, the effects of which have not stabilized, or has not synchronized the timing of medication to coincide with mealtimes. Optimal times differ for individuals. Some find that the swallowing improves during an 'on' stage, whilst others report more success when 'off' because of concurring dyskinetic movements associated with medication. Observation of the swallow should include both liquid and solid consistencies, with the therapist monitoring for any of the characteristics outlined above. Consideration has to be given to three areas in particular: airway protection, nutritional requirements and hydration.

Cervical auscultation

Some therapists will use cervical auscultation as an adjunct to assessment of the swallow. Using a stethoscope held against the neck at the junction of the cricothyroid cartilage and the trachea, the therapist listens for abnormal breath or swallow coordination sounds.

Pulse oximetry

This is another useful tool that may be used. In this case, the oxygen saturation of the blood stream is measured by a probe attached to the fingertip, before, during and after swallowing. Respiratory rate will commonly increase and the percentage of oxygen in the blood will fall if aspiration is occurring.

Videofluoroscopy

Videofluoroscopy or a 'modified barium swallow' is performed on some people with PD. This allows the therapist to ascertain the risk of aspiration, the benefit of one therapeutic strategy over another and the most conducive consistency for the individual to swallow. However, for some people with PD there may be factors that hinder or exclude these benefits. It is crucial for the referring party to consider whether the person with PD can:

- Maintain sitting balance for approximately 15 minutes
- Maintain appropriate levels of alertness for the duration
- Tolerate the potentially stressful environment in which it takes place
- Replicate a natural swallow in a false environment
- Act on recommended swallow strategies on command
- Coordinate medication to coincide with either the desired 'on' or 'off' stage

Clearly, the therapist needs to consider whether an individual's management would change as a result of the videofluoroscopy and whether exposure to radiation is warranted.

Fibreoptic endoscopic evaluation of swallowing safety (FEESS)

In FEESS, a nasoendoscope is passed down through the nose into the pharynx and is positioned above the larynx. It allows the therapist to view the larynx and pharynx directly while the person is swallowing food and drink. Penetration of food or fluid into the laryngeal vestibule, aspiration below the level of the vocal folds and pooling of material can then be observed. Generally, if marked dyskinesia is present, this assessment is inappropriate.

Treatment of swallowing disorders

Explanation

Explanation of the normal swallow and the effect of PD on the swallow are valuable in increasing an individual's awareness. Rationales for subsequent treatment can be given through models and/or pictures of the oral cavity, pharynx and larynx.

Exercises

Depending on the specific nature of the swallowing disorder, the therapist may provide exercises for the individual with PD to maintain optimal function. Where possible these exercises often focus on the range of movement in the tongue, lips and/or larynx.

Manoeuvres

Some specific swallow manoeuvres have also been found to assist particular difficulties with swallowing in this patient population. The Mendelsohn manoeuvre was designed to increase the extent and duration of laryngeal elevation after the swallow in order to increase the width and duration of cricopharyngeal opening. Effortful breath-holding is intended to increase posterior motion of the tongue base and thus improve bolus clearance from the valleculae.

Compensatory strategies

Compensatory strategies can be taught to individuals with PD in order to help regulate the control and flow of food and fluid. They can result in less of a physical and cognitive burden being placed on the individual with PD and subsequently reduce levels of fatigue. They can include:

- Postural changes. Altering the position of the head using the 'chin tuck' technique whereby the individual consciously lowers the chin towards the chest before swallowing
- Sensory awareness. Increasing sensory awareness can be achieved through increasing the downward pressure of the spoon onto the tongue as the bolus is placed in the oral cavity or providing a bolus with increased sensory characteristics, e.g. a strong distinctive flavour

- Modifications in food presentation. Modifying the volume and speed of food presentation can increase the swallow safety. People with PD often require a smaller bolus and extra time to repeat the swallow in order to clear residue in the pharynx
- Changes in food or fluid consistency and temperature. Changes to the food or fluid consistency may be suggested. These suggestions are generally made to patients with PD when motor skills preclude postural changes, cognitive impairment precludes the use of swallow manoeuvres and/or sensory impairment is so severe that awareness training is not feasible. It is often recommended that fluids should be thickened to either a mildly (as in tomato juice), moderately, (as in a thin yoghurt) or very (as in custard) thick consistency. Modifying the diet to soft options (such as pasta), soft/smooth (such as mashed potato) or puree may also be recommended. A chilled bolus, by stimulating the sensory receptors in the oral cavity, may trigger a swallow response more promptly
- Prompting. External verbal or written prompting to swallow and reducing environmental distractions can be beneficial to some patients who, for cognitive reasons, need to be reminded to swallow

Self versus assisted feeding

Kinaesthetic feedback, obtained through the action of bolus placement, assists in the swallowing process. Self-feeding is therefore advocated whenever possible. It is recommended that when an individual overfills the oral cavity, the size of the bolus is controlled by a carer loading the spoon or fork before handing it to the individual.

The role of the multidisciplinary team

Collaboration with other members of the multidisciplinary team can be valuable in the overall treatment of swallowing disorders. The Parkinson's disease Nurse Specialist will have important knowledge of the medications and their timing required by the individual with PD. Where the swallow is impaired, possibilities of alternative means of administering medication, such as dispersible tablets, liquids, injections or pumps, can be discussed. The physiotherapist will be able to advise on appropriate postural positions and is essential, particularly where the individual runs a high risk of aspiration, in monitoring chest status and the detection of bronchopneumonia. The occupational therapist can make valuable contributions with regard to optimal seating, aids for supported limb mobility and utensils to assist eating and drinking such as the 'Flexicup', Pat Saunders Straw and adapted cutlery. Where a patient has weight loss and is not meeting nutritional and hydration requirements, it is essential that early referral be made to the dietician who can provide information regarding how to achieve and maintain sufficient energy intake. Dieticians may recommend oral supplements or supplements delivered by other means such as a naso-gastric or gastrostomy feeding tube.

Drooling

Drooling occurs where there is an impaired swallow, the characteristics of which are outlined above, and results in pooling of saliva in the oral cavity. Patients with PD often report discomfort and embarrassment and can suffer further complications such as angular cheilitis (sore cracks in the corners of the mouth) due to candidal infection (Marks et al 2001a).

Drooling can be treated through a number of medical procedures, including radiotherapy and botulinum toxin injections to the sublingual, submandibular and parotid glands. Radiotherapy to the parotid salivary gland, however, leads to a permanently dry mouth and can cause irreversible damage to the blood vessels of the bone in the irradiated area. Botulinum injections are a relatively newer treatment, but their effects are not permanent, lasting up to approximately 3 months.

Recently, people with PD have found success with an intervention programme based on behaviour modification (Marks et al 2001b). The programme aims to increase awareness of the swallow mechanism in order to provide more control over drooling. This is done through explanations of how and where saliva is produced, the function of saliva, the normal swallow mechanism and why drooling occurs. The intervention also requires the individual to complete swallow frequency charts at home and to practise swallows following an auditory cue from a swallow reminder brooch, specifically designed to emit intermittent bleeps. (Photocopiable charts are available from Marks and Rainbow 2001.)

Key points

- People with PD inevitably suffer the consequences of impaired communication and swallowing
- Speech and language therapists depend on the multidisciplinary team to ensure that best practice is followed; the nursing staff play a crucial, often pivotal, role within the team
- Management of communication and swallowing needs to be patient-focused if it is to be successful, as progress will be made only through listening to the individual

Acknowledgement

To Lizzie Marks, Chief Speech and Language Therapist, The Middlesex Hospital, for her energy, enthusiasm and support in the field of communication and swallowing difficulties in people with Parkinson's disease.

Useful addresses

Further advice and handouts regarding communication and swallowing
Parkinson's Disease Society of the United Kingdom, 215 Vauxhall Bridge Road, London SW1V 1EJ. Tel 020 7931 8080 or e-mail to mailbox@pdsuk.demon.co.uk

The Frenchay Dysarthria Assessment
(Pamela Enderby 1980) Available from College Hill Press, San Diego.

The Assessment of Intelligibility of Dysarthric Speech
(Yorkston and Beukleman, 1981).
Taskmaster Limited, Morris Road, Leicester LE2 6BR.

Lightwriter Communication Aids
Toby Churchill Limited, 20 Panton Street, Cambridge CB2 IHP.
Tel. 01223 576117

Voice Amplifier
Available from Lions Club International.
David Lloyd, Lions Speech Aid, 3 Campbell Close, Buckingham MK18 7HP, Bucks. Tel/Fax 01280 813747 or e-mail dave@lloydo5.freeserve.co.uk
and
Kapitex Healthcare Limited, Kapitex House, 1 Sandbeck Way, Wetherby, West Yorkshire LS22 7GH. Tel 01937 580211

The 'Flexicup'
Kapitex Healthcare Ltd (see above).

Pat Saunders Straw
Nottingham Rehab supplies, 17 Ludlow Hill Road, Melton Road, West Bridgford, Nottingham NG2 6HD.

Swallow reminder brooch
Winslow Health and Rehabilitation, Goyt Side Road, Chesterfield, Derbyshire S40 2PH. Tel 08459211777 email sales@winslow-cat.com

References

Berry W R (1983) Treatment of hypokinetic dysarthria. In: Dysarthria and Apraxia, Current Therapy of Communication Disorders. New York: Thieme-Stratton pp. 91–99.

Dooneief G, Mirabello E, Bell K, Marder K, Stern Y and Mayeux R (1992) An estimate of the incidence of depression in idiopathic Parkinson's disease. Archives of Neurology 49(3): 305–307.

Enderby P (1980) The Frenchay Dysarthria Assessment. San Diego: College Hill Press.

Johnson J A and Pring T R (1990) Speech therapy and Parkinson's disease: a review and further data. British Journal of Disorders of Communication 25: 183–194.

Klasner ER and Yorkston K M (2000) AAC for Huntington disease and Parkinson's disease, planning for change. In: R Beukelman, K M Yorkston and J Reichle (eds.) Augmentative and Alternative Communication for Adults with Acquired Neurologic Disorders. Baltimore: Paul Brookes Publishing pp. 233–270.

Leopald N and Kagel M (1996) Prepharyngeal dysphagia in Parkinson's disease. Dysphagia 11: 14–22.

Logemann J A (1998) Evaluation and Treatment of Swallowing Disorders. Austin: Pro.ed Publishers. Available from Winslow Press.

Longstreth W, Nelson L, Linde M and Munoz D (1992) Utility of sickness impact profile in Parkinson's disease. Journal of Geriatric Psychiatry and Neurology 5(3): 142–148.

Marigliani C, Gates S and Jacks D (1998) Speech pathology and Parkinson's disease. Chapter 7 in: M Morris and R Iansek (eds.) Parkinson's Disease: A Team Approach. Melbourne: Southern Healthcare Network.

Marks L, Hyland K M and Fiske J (2001a) Oral considerations: communication and swallowing problems, diet and oral care. In: J R Playfer and J V Hindle (eds.) Parkinson's Disease in the Older Patient. London: Arnold Publishers pp. 134–163.

Marks L and Rainbow D (2001) Working with Dysphagia. Bicester: Winslow Press.

Marks L, Turner K, O'Sullivan J, Deighton B and Lees A (2001b) Drooling in Parkinson's disease: a novel speech and language therapy intervention. International Journal of Language and Communication Disorders 36(Suppl): 282–287.

Murdoch B E (1998) Dysarthria. A Physiological Approach to Assessment and Treatment. Cheltenham: Nelson Thornes Publishers Ltd.

Oxtoby M (1982) Parkinson's Disease Patients and their Social Needs. London: Parkinson's Disease Society.

Ramig L A, Bonitati C M, Lemke J H and Horii Y (1994) Voice treatment for patients with Parkinson's disease: development of an approach and preliminary efficacy data. Journal of Medical Speech–Language Pathology 2: 191–209.

Ramig L, Pawlas A and Countryman S (1995) The Lee Silverman Voice Treatment. Iowa City, IA: National Centre for Voice and Speech.

Scott S (1998) Parkinson's Disease Speech and Language Therapy Pack. London: Parkinson's Disease Society of the United Kingdom.

Scott S and Caird F (1983) Speech therapy for Parkinson's disease. Journal of Neurology, Neurosurgery and Psychiatry 46(2): 140–144.

Scott S, Caird F and Willims B (1985) Communication in Parkinson's Disease. London: Croom Helm.

Yorkston K M and Beukleman R (1981) The Assessment of Intelligibility of Dysarthric Speech. Leicester: Taskmaster Limited.

Chapter ten

Affective disorders in Parkinson's disease

CAROLYN NOBLE

Introduction

When faced with living with a degenerative, progressive condition such as Parkinson's disease (PD), people are very likely to experience emotional and psychological difficulties linked with various stages in its progression. Primarily this is associated with acceptance and adjustment to the initial diagnosis and anxiety relating to uncertainties regarding the progression of the condition. Fluctuations in mood, low self-esteem and lack of confidence can increase anxiety and depression, and these may result in a gradual withdrawal from social situations. This withdrawal can lead to changes in relationships, loss of friends, poor self-esteem and increased dependency on health and social care networks. Early recognition of emotional and psychological problems can reduce disability and dependency on others.

Treatment can be complex, as the nature of affective disorders may be influenced by biological, psychological and pharmacological factors. Medication and psychotherapies may be used independently or in combination and, for anxiety disorders, cognitive therapy may be the preferred treatment option (Whitworth and Waterfall 1997). This chapter will discuss anxiety and depression in PD and will briefly describe the various treatment options currently available.

Depression and anxiety are commonly linked with PD and there has been much debate over the evidence suggesting an organic or a reactive aetiology. These frequently co-exist and may have a major impact on quality of life. In contrast with the general elderly population, depression and panic disorder are commonly observed, and anxiety disorders, particularly generalized anxiety, panic disorder and social phobia, occur in higher rates in people with PD than in other disease comparison populations (Hegeman et al 1996).

Anxiety

Anxiety is a state characterized by a vague and unpleasant sense of apprehension often accompanied by autonomic symptoms, such as palpitations and dry mouth. Anxiety may serve as a beneficial alerting signal that can warn of impending danger and stimulate the taking of appropriate measures, but it may also be pathological if the symptoms are excessive or if they occur at inappropriate times (Hegeman et al 1996).

Studies have shown that anxiety symptoms in PD usually appear after the diagnosis is received (Henderson et al 1992) and this is commonly associated with the difficulties experienced in acknowledging and adjusting to the information. Several studies have stressed the importance of the need to understand how individual people experience and adapt to this illness (Dakof et al 1986). A study by MacCarthy and Brown (1989) explored the relationships between aspects of psychological adjustment (depression, positive affect and acceptance of illness) and physical illness (duration and stage of illness and functional disability). The study revealed that self-esteem, coping style and practical support contributed significantly to the variance in psychological adjustment.

Presentations of anxiety

Anxiety in PD may present in a number of ways including:

- Generalized anxiety disorder
- Panic disorder
- Social phobia
- Obsessive compulsive disorder

Generalized anxiety disorder (GAD)

The individual experiences pervasive anxiety because their beliefs about themselves and the environment make them prone to interpret a wide range of situations in a threatening way. Issues around GAD usually revolve around acceptance, competence, responsibility, control and the symptoms of anxiety themselves (Beck 1985).

Acceptance

For people with PD there may be concerns about feeling accepted by others who may not be aware of their difficulties or who may have misinterpreted or failed to understand the symptoms. The 'core belief' of the person concerned with acceptance is that they may be flawed in some way and this may be unacceptable to others. These beliefs can result in fears of rejection and will directly affect self-esteem. This person is afraid that others will notice their flaws and, because other peoples' opinions directly affect self-esteem, they are highly dependent on feedback from others. They may exaggerate the extent and significance of social acceptance and rejection and believe everyone's acceptance essential and equally important.

Competence

As the condition progresses the individual may experience difficulties in performing certain tasks because of the limitations imposed by the symptoms and may feel less competent or less able. For someone who has anxiety centred around 'competency', their main belief may involve feelings of inferiority. This may result in the person feeling unsure of themselves and social skills and abilities may be minimized or overlooked.

Control

When faced with significant life changes, such as being diagnosed with a chronic progressive illness, individuals can experience feelings of 'loss of control' over their lives. Anxiety based on core beliefs involving 'control' suggests that the person is being dominated by others or events outside that person's control. In the past this person may have been in a situation where they perceived themselves as having 'little or no control', e.g. having a domineering parent.

Responsibility

Reversal of roles within a partnership or within families may create feelings of anxiety as responsibilities change and the individual becomes more dependent on others. For those with core beliefs involving dependency or incompetence there may be problems around dealing with day-to-day responsibilities. This person may rely excessively for help in decision-making and initiating new tasks.

The symptoms of anxiety

These can generate further anxiety, usually because the symptoms have been misinterpreted.

Panic disorder

Individuals experience panic attacks because they have an enduring tendency to interpret a range of bodily sensations in a catastrophic way. For example, palpitations, breathlessness and dizziness during a panic attack can be misinterpreted as indications of impending disaster, such as heart attack, collapse, fainting or loss of control (Beck 1985).

Social phobia

Social phobia centres around negative evaluation, criticism or rejection by other people and may focus on particular aspects of social interactions such as speaking or eating in public.

Obsessive compulsive disorder

Obsessions are unwanted and intrusive thoughts, images or urges which are difficult for the individual to dismiss and usually trigger obsessive behaviours to reduce anxiety, such as 'checking', compulsive cleaning or washing, and ritualistic routines.

Development of anxiety disorders in PD

As the motor symptoms of PD become increasingly evident, individual responses to these changes vary considerably from mild embarrassment to a gradual withdrawal from social activities, which may lead to the development of social phobia. However, Lauterbach and Duvoisin (1992) noted that a study of people diagnosed with social phobia revealed anxiety symptoms even before the diagnosis. This would suggest that anxiety symptoms could be due to neurobiological processes occurring in PD and not simply to psychosocial factors related to the impact of the diagnosis. There is no indication why some individuals have a greater tendency to develop anxiety-related symptoms, but this may be related to previous experiences in that person's life.

Worries, fears and anxieties affect us all differently and understanding aspects of life that may make the individual susceptible to such problems can enable that person to manage and prevent further problems occurring. Listening to the person with PD and reviewing their personal history may reveal certain risk factors which may predispose the individual to the development of anxiety-related problems.

Risk factors

Personality type

- A competitive person may have fears of failing and may relate having their condition to being 'less than perfect'
- An ambitious person or someone who is a perfectionist may have difficulties with feelings of 'control' or 'lack of control' over events
- A worrier usually develops an easily triggered stress response
- Low self-esteem can result in the person feeling as though in some way they may 'deserve' what is happening to them and this can be associated with 'guilt'

Family history

- Assumptions about the self formed during childhood can influence the idiosyncratic meaning of an event

- There may be familial links with anxiety and depression predisposing development of similar problems in the individual

Life stressors

- Significant events such as financial problems, job insecurity or relationship difficulties can result in anxiety
- 'Clustering' of life events, e.g. marriage and a house move, together with job change, can make the individual more vulnerable to stress

Psychological style – 'catastrophizing'

- Jumping to the wrong conclusions
- Biaised thinking, i.e. paying more attention to the negative and ignoring positive aspects

Poor coping styles

- Avoidance of the problem by 'keeping busy' in contrast to using problem-solving as a practical way of dealing with problems
- Using distraction as a way of not confronting or paying attention to the problem
- Misuse of drugs and alcohol

Social support

- Emotional problems increase with lower levels of social support

Motor symptoms

It has been reported that people with PD who experience unpredictable motor fluctuations experience higher levels of anxiety (Henderson et al 1992; Menza et al 1993). Whilst most studies report a degree of worsening of anxiety levels in the 'off' state, Menza et al (1990) revealed an improvement in mood or anxiety from the 'off' to the 'on' state followed by a worsening of anxiety in the 'on' state when dyskinesias returned. This would suggest that behavioural responses probably represent an emotional reaction to the motor symptoms. However, changes in levels of the neurotransmitters serotonin and noradrenaline may precipitate anxiety and panic attacks (Vazquez et al 1993). In addition, a worsening of symptoms during periods of high anxiety, during which symptoms are not well controlled by anti-PD medication, is frequently recognized.

Treatment for anxiety disorders

Medication is not recommended for every anxiety disorder and may even cause a worsening of symptoms for people with PD. The perceived benefits must be measured against side-effect profiles and individual circumstances (Andrews and Jenkins 1999). A wide variety of drugs is used to treat anxiety in PD including selective serotonin reuptake inhibitors (SSRIs), beta-blockers and tricyclics.

SSRIs (e.g. fluoxetine, sertraline, paroxetine) may be effective for suppression of panic but generally higher doses are required to treat anxiety than for depression and it may take longer to experience an improvement in symptoms. Beta-blockers can be used when performance anxiety is the main problem and may reduce anxiety and distress by minimizing or preventing noticeable symptoms of anxiety, such as tremor. Tricyclic antidepressants are helpful in the treatment of depression, panic disorder, obsessive compulsive disorder and chronic pain syndrome. However, the anticholinergic effect may cause problems, particularly for elderly people.

Psychotherapies introduced with or without medication may be the treatment of choice. Brown and Jahanshashi (1995a) suggest that a psychotherapy programme should be adapted for individuals and caregivers throughout the course of the illness. Evidence for psychotherapy treatment modalities is somewhat limited. However, some studies have explored the effect of cognitive therapy on young people with PD (Dreisig et al 1999); for social phobia in PD (Heinrichs et al 2001); coping styles (Sanders-Dewey et al 2001); adjustment to PD (Speer 1993; McQuillen 1998; Gilbar and Harel 2000) and psychosocial factors in PD (MacCarthy and Brown 1989).

Cognitive behavioural therapy (CBT)

The aim of cognitive therapy is to enable the person to bring about desired changes in their life through the process of cognitive change. These changes can be brought about by challenging beliefs and negative thoughts which affect the way in which the person perceives or misinterprets problems.

Looking at problems or situations from a different perspective can often lead to new conclusions and opportunities to explore new solutions or approaches. Cognitive therapy is not about 'thinking more positively', as this may lead to important signals being missed. It is a way of allowing some flexibility into thought processes to encourage more helpful responses and coping patterns to stressful situations.

It could be argued that people faced with the experience of living with PD may indeed have realistic negative thoughts and these may be a natural response to stress and part of the process of grieving. If the process of adjustment is ongoing it may not necessarily be appropriate for the individual to undergo a course of cognitive therapy. What is important is early identification of perceived uncertainty and psychological distress in order for the individual to receive guidance from a professional who can provide information about the condition and the management of associated symptoms (Sanders-Dewey et al 2001). This could include identification of coping styles, coping strategies and support networks. Information about the condition can be provided in written form, by referral to appropriate professionals or by facilitating introductions to others who have been similarly diagnosed and are now managing their condition well.

CBT strategies

The cognitive therapist may use some of the following strategies:

- Explore the advantages versus the disadvantages of negative thinking. Use the negative thoughts to prompt problem solving, for example: 'You may be unable to carry out this activity in the same way that you have always done but have you considered different ways of achieving the same goal?' Realistic negative thoughts can be part of the normal process of adjustment, but they can disrupt a person's life if they are repetitive or ruminative
- Look at ways that ruminative thoughts can affect the individual's ability to enjoy areas of their life that are open to them and the ways in which relationships can be affected if the ruminations become destructive
- Ask the patient to record negative thoughts as this can determine how much time is devoted to unconstructive thinking versus the time available for constructive engagement with life. When the individual realizes how much time is being wasted in this way, they may be willing to attempt distraction techniques
- Employ distraction techniques:
  - Activity scheduling – this is a way of gradually introducing increasing amounts of activity during the day
  - Scheduling time for worry or grieving, i.e. negotiate specific time slots which can only be taken up with negative thoughts or worrying. If negative thoughts creep in at other times the person would be encouraged to 'block' the thoughts or distract themselves by engaging in an activity
  - Find an area of life that may be controlled which instills a feeling of overall control. Encourage activities which help that person to feel that they are contributing

Depression

Depression occurs in 40–50% of people diagnosed with PD (Doonief et al 1992), 20% of whom will meet the criteria for major depression and the remainder will display a number of symptoms related to anxiety and depression (Starkstein et al 1989). Not surprisingly, this can have a major impact on quality of life. A recent study by Herlofsen et al (1999) revealed that depression was one of the most detrimental factors which affected the quality of life of people with PD. Horn (1974) suggested that people with PD exhibit more symptoms of depression than other age- and gender-matched people diagnosed with other chronic conditions including rheumatoid arthritis, paraplegia and cerebrovascular accident (stroke).

Kremer and Starkstein (2000) suggest that most people with PD may eventually develop depression at some point during the progression of the condition. They also indicate a significantly faster decline in activities of daily living and cognitive functioning with major depression and a faster progression along the stages of the illness compared with non-depressed people with PD.

A number of studies have explored the relationship between age of onset of PD and the frequency of depression. Cole et al (1996) reported twice the frequency of depression in younger people with PD. People with early onset PD are particularly vulnerable to depression as a reaction to the illness and the detrimental effect on their careers, financial security and quality of life during their most productive years (Taylor and Saint-Cyr 1990). The early onset of PD causes 'premature social ageing' whereby the level of social handicap is inconsistent with the patient's age and may further contribute to the risk factors for depression (Brown and Jahanshashi 1995b).

Depression is a mood state that is characterized by significantly lowered mood and a loss of interest or pleasure in activities that are normally enjoyable. It may be mild, moderate or severe. Symptoms of depression may include:

- Depressed mood
- Disturbed appetite
- Fearfulness linked with social withdrawal
- Delusions and hallucinations
- Reduced energy and reduced activity
- Decreased libido
- Disturbed sleep and early waking
- Recurring unpleasant thoughts
- Loss of interest or enjoyment
- Reduced concentration and attention
- Reduced self-esteem and self-confidence
- Feelings of guilt or worthlessness
- Fatigue

Psychological factors such as personality, coping strategies and social resources are thought to influence the degree of severity of depression in

PD (Brown and Jahanshashi 1995b). Depression seems to be the single most important factor associated with the severity of dementia, and early antidepressant treatment seems to decrease cognitive decline in depressed people with PD (Starkstein et al 1989; Valldeoriola et al 1997).

Recognizing depression in PD

The symptoms of PD share many of the features commonly observed in affective disorders and this contributes to the problems of recognizing and diagnosing depression. The DSM-IV (Diagnostic and Statistical Manual for Mental Disorders, American Psychiatric Association 1994) criteria for the diagnosis of depression include anhedonia or depressed mood for more than 2 weeks together with at least five of the following symptoms:

- Significant weight change
- Insomnia or hypersomnia
- Agitation and psychomotor retardation
- Decreased concentration and indecisiveness
- Recurrent thoughts of death or suicide ideation
- Feelings of worthlessness or inappropriate guilt
- Fatigue/loss of energy

Some of these symptoms can occur in the non-depressed person with PD. Assessment of mood can be obtained by the use of a standardized depression scale such as the Beck Depression Inventory (BDI) (Beck et al 1961), or the Geriatric Depression Screening Scale (Yesavage et al 1983). Once diagnosed, the depression should be treated promptly to reduce distress, improve quality of life and prevent further cognitive decline.

Treatment options for depression

Treatment will involve some or all of the following:

- Assessment (Hospital Anxiety and Depression Scale (HADS) (Snaith and Zigmond 1983), BDI, Geriatric Depression Scale)
- Education and support for the individual and the family. Depression is an illness, not a 'weakness' and can be treated effectively if recognized early on. The rate of recurrence is high, so the signs and symptoms should be reported quickly in times of relapse
- Reduce associated problems – structure problem-solving, improve sleep pattern, increase activity, relaxation training, assertiveness training and interpersonal skills training
- Psychotherapy
- Medication

- Prevent relapse or recurrence of depression (CBT strategies)
- Electroconvulsive therapy (ECT) has been reported to improve mood and motor symptoms in PD (Moellentine et al 1998).

Antidepressant medication

Antidepressant medication needs to be considered carefully against the less favourable side effects which may potentially worsen PD symptoms. The choice of antidepressant will depend on the following:

- Its symptom profile, e.g. a sedative antidepressant may be helpful if insomnia is a problem
- Side effects (e.g. avoid anticholinergic drugs in the treatment of elderly people)
- Co-morbid medical problems (e.g. avoid anticholinergic drugs in people with glaucoma)
- Existing medications and possible drug interactions
- The individual's current or past responses to medication

If the individual develops psychotic depression with delusions and hallucinations, antipsychotic medication should be added to the antidepressant medication during the active phase of treatment.

Response to antidepressant treatment varies but it may be 2–3 weeks before an effect is noticed and 4–8 weeks before the full antidepressant effect occurs. However, some symptoms, such as insomnia, may respond in a shorter period of time. Antidepressant treatment is usually continued for 6–12 months after recovery from the first episode or longer for people who have had two or more severe episodes of depression. Medication should always be withdrawn gradually. Relapse can occur after medication is stopped, so careful monitoring is needed to help to detect signs of relapse early (Andrews and Jenkins 1999). For people with moderate to severe depression it is advisable to involve the community psychiatric nurse and team.

Conclusion

Nurses can make a difference to people who are experiencing affective disorders in PD as they can aid in early recognition of affective disorders. Patients who are suspected to be experiencing anxiety or depression should be encouraged to discuss their problems with either their general practitioner or neurologist who in turn can initiate prompt treatment. Nurses should consider:

- Using clinical assessment tools such as the HADS to aid in early identification of affective disorders. HADS is very quick and easy to administer

and provides an indication of mood and levels of anxiety. Alternatively, the BDI could be used; this is longer than the HADS, but it is relatively easy to administer
- Improving their professional knowledge and understanding of affective disorders. This can be done by:
  - Developing links with community psychiatric nurses, psychotherapists and clinical psychologists. Exchange information about roles to help improve services for people with PD experiencing affective disorders
  - Finding out if further training is available in basic counselling skills or more in-depth training in psychotherapies including cognitive behaviour therapy (CBT) or cognitive analytical therapy (CAT). It is not necessary to come from a mental health training background to access these courses and they may influence the way in which the nurse develops professionally

Key points

- Depression and anxiety disorders occur in higher rates in people with PD than in normal or other disease comparison populations
- Early recognition of psychological and emotional difficulties can help to reduce disability or dependency on others
- Most people with PD may develop depression at some point during the progression of the condition
- There may be a significantly faster decline in activities of daily living and cognitive functioning with major depression and a faster progression along the stages of the illness compared with non-depressed people with the condition
- Early assessment, education, support and treatment are essential and treatment can be effective, although the rate of recurrence of affective disorders is high
- CBT may be the preferred treatment option, or it may be used with medication
- There is a range of treatment options for affective disorders, however more research needs to be carried out for a definitive framework of management of affective disorders in PD

References

American Psychiatric Association, committee of nomenclature and statistics (1994) Diagnostic and Statistical Manual of Mental Disorders (DSM-IV). Washington DC: American Psychiatric Association.

Andrews G and Jenkins R (eds.) (1999) Management of Mental Disorders (UK Edition). Sydney: World Health Organization Collaborating Centre for Mental Health and Substance Abuse.

Beck A T, Ward C H, Mendelson M, Mock J and Erbaugh J (1961) An inventory for measuring depression. Archives of General Psychiatry 4: 561–571.

Beck A T (1985) Anxiety Disorders and Phobias. A cognitive perspective. New York: Guilford Press.

Brown R and Jahanshashi M (1995a) Depression in Parkinson's disease: a psychosocial viewpoint. In: W J Weiner and A E Long (eds.) Advances in Neurology, volume 65. Behavioural Neurology of Movement Disorders. New York: Raven Press pp. 61–84.

Brown R and Jahanshashi M (1995b) Depression in Parkinson's disease: a psychological viewpoint. Advances in Neurology 65: 61–84.

Cole S A, Woodard J L, Juncos J L, Kogos J L, Youngstrom E A and Watts R L (1996) Depression and disability in Parkinson's disease. Journal of Neuropsychiatry and Clinical Neurosciences 8: 20–25.

Dakof A U, Gayle A and Mendelsohn G A (1986) Parkinson's disease: the psychological aspects of chronic illness. American Psychological Association Bulletin 99(3): 375–387.

Doonief G, Mirabello E, Bell K, Marder K, Stern Y and Mayeux R (1992) An estimate of the incidence of depression in idiopathic Parkinson's. Archives of Neurology 49: 305–307.

Dreisig H, Beckmann J, Wermuth L, Skoulund S and Beck P (1999) Psychological effects of structured cognitive psychotherapy in young patients with Parkinson's Disease. A pilot study. Nordic Journal of Psychiatry 53(3): 217–221.

Gilbar O and Harel Y (2000) Adjustment to Parkinson's disease by patients and their spouses. Illness, Crisis and Loss 8(1): 47–59.

Hegeman R I, Schiffer R B and Kurlan R (1996) Anxiety and Parkinson's disease. Journal of Neuropsychiatry 8: 383–392.

Heinrichs N, Hoffman E C and Hoffman S G (2001) Cognitive-behavioral treatment for social phobia in Parkinson's disease: a single case study. Cognitive and Behavioral Practice 8(4): 328–335.

Herlofsen K K, Larsen J P and Tandberg E (1999) Influence of clinical and demographic variables on quality of life in patients with Parkinson's disease. Journal of Neurology, Neurosurgery and Psychiatry 66: 431–435.

Henderson R, Kurlan R, Kersun J M and Como P (1992) Preliminary examination of the comorbidity of anxiety and depression in Parkinson's disease. Journal of Neuropsychiatry and Clinical Neurosciences 4:257–264

Horn S (1974) Psychological factors in parkinsonism. Journal of Neurology, Neurosurgery and Psychiatry 36: 925–935.

Kremer J and Starkstein S E (2000) Affective disorders in Parkinson's disease. International Review of Psychiatry 12: 290–297.

Lauterbach E C, Duvoisin R C (1992) Anxiety disorders in familial parkinsonism (letter). American Journal of Psychiatry 148: 274.

MacCarthy B and Brown R (1989) Some psychological factors in Parkinson's disease. British Journal of Clinical Psychology 28(1): 41–52.

McQuillen A D (1998) The role of coping goals in adaptation to Parkinson's disease. Dissertation Abstracts International: Section B: The Sciences and Engineering 58: 7–13.

Menza M A, Sage J, Marshall E, Cody R and Duvoisin R G (1990) Mood changes and 'on/off' phenomena in Parkinson's disease. Movement Disorders 5: 148–151.

Menza M A, Robertson-Hoffman D E and Bonapace A S (1993) Parkinson's disease and anxiety: comorbidity with depression. Biological Psychiatry 34: 465–470.

Moellentine C, Rummans T, Ahlskog J E, Harmsen W S, Suman V J, O'Connor M K and Black J L (1998) Effectiveness of ECT in patients with parkinsonism. Journal of Neuropsychiatry 10: 187–193.

Sanders-Dewey A V, Neva E J, Mullins L L and Chaney J M (2001) Coping style, perceived uncertainty in illness and distress in individuals with Parkinson's disease and their caregivers. Rehabilitation Psychology 46(40): 363–381.

Snaith R P and Zigmond A S (1983) Hospital Anxiety and Depression Scale. Acta Psychiatrica Scandinavica 67: 361–370.

Speer D C (1993) Predicting Parkinson's disease patient and caregiver adjustment: preliminary findings. Behaviour, Health and Ageing 3(3): 139–146.

Starkstein S E and Kremer J (2000) Affective disorders in Parkinson's disease. International Review of Psychiatry 12: 290–297.

Starkstein S E, Preziosi T J, Berthier M L, Buldoc P L, Mayberg H S and Robinson R G (1989) Depression and cognitive impairment in Parkinson's disease. Brain 112: 1141–1153.

Taylor A E and Saint-Cyr J A (1990) Depression in Parkinson's disease: reconciling physiological and psychological perspectives. Journal of Neuropsychiatry and Clinical Neurosciences 2: 92–98.

Valldeoriola F A, Nobbe A and Tolosa E (1997) Treatment of behavioural disturbances in Parkinson's disease. Journal of Neural Transmission 51(suppl): 175–204.

Vazquez A, Jimenez-Jimenez F J, Garcia-Ruiz P and Garcia-Urra D (1993) Panic attacks in Parkinson's disease: a long term complication of levodopa therapy. Acta Neurologica Scandinavica 87:14–18.

Yesavage J, Brink L L, Rose T L, Lum O, Huang V, Adey M B and Leirer V O (1983) Development and validation of a geriatric depression screening scale: a preliminary report. Journal of Psychiatric Research 17: 37–49.

Whitworth F and Waterfall M (1997) Chapter 4. In: R Iansek and M Morris (eds.) Parkinson's Disease: a Team Approach. Blackburn Australia: Buscombe Vicprint Ltd.

CHAPTER ELEVEN

Assessing the needs of people with Parkinson's disease

JACQUI HANDLEY

The aim of this chapter is to highlight the range and depth of problems that a person with Parkinson's disease (PD) may experience and the assessments that will be required throughout the course of the disease. Parkinson's disease is a challenging chronic illness that, in time, is likely to affect most aspects of daily living. Many patients have difficulty explaining the exact nature of their problems and an informed assessor can help patients identify priorities and set realistic goals for treatment. Nurses are well placed to complete such comprehensive assessments, working in conjunction with the multidisciplinary team. At present there is no comprehensive, yet user-friendly, assessment tool available but, taking a quality of life approach and adapting some of the tools that are available, an informed team can make effective assessments of need. Whatever tools are chosen, they should lead the clinician to ask appropriate questions and allow the patient and carer to tell their story.

Introduction

Contemporary literature seems to agree that PD is a much more complex illness than purely a disorder of movement. James Parkinson (1817) gave his name to the disease when he recorded his observations of patients with tremor and gait disturbances. He used the term 'the shaking palsy', or paralysis agitans, and, until recently, PD was viewed primarily as a movement disorder. However, PD is now recognized as a chronic progressive neuropsychiatric disorder, which may also affect cognitive processes, emotions and autonomic function.

Individual experiences of PD will vary widely according to age, disease duration, concurrent ill health, lifestyle, social situation and inherent personality. An assessment of need must therefore focus on building a comprehensive picture of the individual's circumstances including their physical, psychological, environmental and social domains (Struck et al 1993).

Meara and coworkers (2001) describe assessment as a process which should be carried out to inform, recognize, measure and evaluate the situation before any decisions are made about interventions or treatment. Many healthcare professionals view assessment as a core, fundamental activity of their role. The process begins immediately and, at times, unconsciously, on contact with a patient, taking in both verbal and non-verbal cues. When this information-gathering stage is complete, the details can then be processed using professional knowledge and expertise to lead to decisions on treatment.

The traditional approach to assessment in PD has focused on motor and movement problems and response to drug therapy. However, Clarke (2001) suggests this narrow focus is inadequate and that assessment in PD should focus on the quality of life of the individual. A quality of life approach takes a broad view to include the individual's perceptions and experiences of the disease (Fitzpatrick and Alonso 1999). As treatments for PD can only relieve rather than cure symptoms, maintaining quality of life is the treatment goal; it seems appropriate, therefore, to apply this approach to assessment.

For patients to perceive such a comprehensive assessment process as worthwhile, it must lead to improvements in the problems which they consider important. Llach and Martin (1999) suggest that, while measurement of biochemical and physiological changes is of interest to clinicians, patients are more interested in how it will make them feel. Conducting an assessment for PD is therefore a complex activity which is perhaps most effective when undertaken by a multidisciplinary team; it is unlikely that any one professional alone will have all the expertise required (Meara et al 2001).

Assessment tools

As interest in improving the management of PD gains momentum, a common question asked is, 'Which is the most suitable assessment tool?' It is widely agreed, however, that at present there is no one tool available which is sufficiently universal and comprehensive to suit all patients, in all situations (Clarke 2001). The search for an effective assessment tool for PD spans at least 40 years and Llach and Martin (1999) suggest that lack of progress may be because of the substantial amount of work and time required. For a tool to become credible and achieve international recognition it must be valid, reliable, sensitive, and user-friendly in practice.

- Validity means the tool facilitates measurement of the factors it was intended to measure

- Reliability means that measurement error is small even when a tool is used by many different assessors in different situations
- Sensitivity means that detection of real and clinically significant change is reflected in the final score over a period of time

There is a wide variety of assessment tools in current use and some examples are shown in Table 11.1. This chapter cannot include a comprehensive critique of all the tools in use, but the frustrations which occur in practice probably arise because none of them fully meets the above criteria.

Table 11.1 Assessment tools commonly used in PD

Name of tool	Components	Advantages	Disadvantages
Unified Parkinson's Disease Rating Scale (UPDRS) (Fahn et al 1987)	Four sections: motor, mental, daily activities and therapy complications	Comprehensive	Time to complete 30–40 minutes
Hoehn and Yahr Staging Scale (Hoehn and Yahr 1967)	Clinical rating scale 1–5	Well recognized	Lacks detail No assessment of cognition, bladder or bowel function and balance
Northwestern University Disability Scales (Canter et al 1992)	5 sections	Quick and simple to complete. Reasonable sensitivity	Lacks detail
Webster's Scale 1968 (Webster 1968)	10 sections	Quick and simple to complete	Lacks detail
Parkinson's Disease Questionnaire (PDQ 39) (Jenkinson et al 1995)	8 domains, 39 questions	Disease-specific quality of life approach. Recognized internationally. Good reliability	Number of questions. Time for completion

A pathway approach

Whilst not designed as an assessment tool, the Paradigm for Disease Management takes a pathway approach to PD, identifying four stages of the disease, classified as diagnosis, maintenance, complex and palliative

(MacMahon and Thomas 1998). Whilst each individual will have a unique experience of PD, there are trends and similarities that can be drawn together into these four core stages. The paradigm is a disease-specific tool and it can be used in local practice as a guide to what needs are likely to arise at what stage. When used with some of the assessment tools available, this can help to inform professionals of the problems likely to be affecting the individual and some of the possible treatment options.

Diagnostic stage

In traditional medicine the journey with any illness begins when the individual recognizes that something is wrong and goes to their general practitioner (GP). The cardinal signs of PD may not be fully developed at this stage, and a definite diagnosis can be many months away. However, nurses will meet people in this stage either in the surgery, in the community or in hospital. The person is aware that something is wrong and may seek out a nurse to discuss the problems further. Whilst the nurse should not confirm or refute the diagnosis as this stage, it is an opportunity to complete a full assessment of the situation and communicate findings to the doctors involved, in order to help the diagnostic process.

The importance of the diagnostic stage to patients was perhaps not fully recognized until the publication of a large study of 2000 people with PD from six different countries (Findlay 2000). This study found that the factors which most influenced a patient's quality of life were depression, current level of optimism, dependence on others and satisfaction with the information given at diagnosis. Although levels of physical disability may be minimal at this stage, Carter and coworkers (1998) describe being diagnosed with PD as a life-altering experience, which threatens all aspects of quality of life. The four-stage approach highlights the importance of this time and the role of the professionals to help patients and their families develop disease awareness, reduce symptoms and distress and lead to acceptance of the diagnosis (MacMahon and Thomas 1998).

Key points

Assessments during the diagnostic stage should include:

- Knowledge and perceptions of the disease
- Ideas and perceptions of disease progression
- Employment issues
- Benefit entitlement
- Driving

Although continuing to drive will not be a problem for most people at this stage, once diagnosed with PD patients must be advised to inform the DVLA and their insurance companies in accordance with current driving licence policy. Lincoln and Radford (1999) suggest that, at present, there is no objective set of reliable criteria against which to judge fitness to drive, but further developments are anticipated in the near future. It is not the remit of nurses to decide whether a patient is fit to drive, but giving patients advice and practical solutions is appropriate. When conducting general assessments, any concerns raised about the patients' driving abilities should be reported to their doctors.

Maintenance stage

The aims of this stage are to relieve morbidity, prevent complications and promote good health. MacMahon (2001) suggests that typically patients with PD will remain at this stage for around 5 years and, if they received the appropriate support and guidance in the diagnostic stage, may be self-caring with the support of their GP. Some areas promote a shared care approach for this stage with a clear action plan, which enables ongoing patient care across organizational boundaries (Hindle 2001). Where Parkinson's disease Nurse Specialists (PDNSs) are available they can take the lead in this as their role usually allows them to work across primary and secondary care boundaries (Morgan and Moran 2001). Such role flexibility is particularly suitable for people with PD who may need assessments of their functioning in a variety of settings such as at home, in the clinic or as an inpatient.

Treatment at this stage aims to promote normal function and self-care and minimize time spent with health professionals. However, a regular assessment programme is necessary to highlight disease progression, review treatments and prevent complications. Regular reviews also provide opportunities for health promotion and to check compliance and understanding of drug regimes. Teaching the principles of drug management to a relatively well patient can be very effective, as shown by Ellgring et al (1993), who found that interventions designed to build long-term coping skills were most effectively taught in early disease. However, Carter (1998) warns that too much education in early disease can prove overwhelming and anxiety-provoking and recommends that patients should only be encouraged to learn about current problems. Perhaps, therefore, another aspect of assessment is that the nurse considers what is the appropriate amount of information for that particular patient and at that particular time.

Key points

Assessments during the maintenance stage should include:

- Promoting normal function
- Regular reviews to monitor disease progression, review treatments and prevent complications
- Education on long-term coping strategies
- Needs for information and support

Complex stage

In terms of physical disability this could be seen as the most difficult stage of PD, as all the symptoms become fully developed and the patient struggles to remain active and independent. Many problems will be multiple and intertwined, and assessments must be sufficiently comprehensive to include all factors relating both to PD and to other health problems. This can result in a huge amount of information, and strategies are needed to analyse what can, and what cannot, be changed. In terms of medications, the complex phase is reached when either five or more doses or more than two different drugs are being used. During the earlier stages most patients find that their medications are effective, well tolerated and very helpful in improving their quality of life; in the complex stage, expectations remain high but the scope of current medicines may prove inadequate. Assessments must, therefore, include helping the patient to set realistic goals for treatment and asking the question 'Which is the worst problem for you at the moment?'

In recent years evidence has mounted that the needs of people with PD have been underestimated and often overlooked (Koplas et al 1999). Knowledge of the complexity and global effects of the disease is developing rapidly, but effective treatments for many of the symptoms are not yet available; a major challenge of the complex stage is managing symptoms versus side effects of treatments.

MacMahon (2001) suggests there are six components to managing PD effectively:

- Education
- Health promotion
- Diet and exercise
- Neurorehabilitative education
- Drugs
- Surgery

An assessment of a person in the complex stage needs to consider all of these approaches in order to meet the patient's many needs. Treatments will require a level of commitment from patients and their family in order to be effective, and it may be necessary to establish what they would like to tackle first.

Most of the care and support for people with PD is provided in the community but occasionally hospital admissions become necessary. This occurs more commonly in the later stages, either to reassess needs and redesign treatments, or to treat concurrent health problems. Unfortunately many patients have a story to tell of a bad experience as an inpatient, with one of the biggest complaints related to poor understanding of their needs by hospital professionals and poor administration of drug regimes. Often admissions are to busy surgical or trauma wards where staff do not specialize in managing people with PD and may not be familiar with the effects of infection or anaesthetics on PD control. When a PDNS is available, education and liaison with hospital staff is a useful part of their role but this can prove difficult with high staff turnover and busy workloads. A structured programme of hospital-wide education on PD can be very helpful to raise awareness and set standards for practice. PD awareness includes knowledge of the four cardinal symptoms and recognition that high levels of pain, fatigue and depression can also occur (Hindle 2001).

When a patient is admitted for assessment and stabilization of PD, all nursing staff should understand the need for detailed assessments of the problems being experienced, 'on/off' cycles and fluctuations, and recording of the response to drug treatments. Assessments are likely to be complex and time-consuming during this stage but must include the patient's normal coping strategies and the recent changes leading to hospital admission. A particular issue is the completion of accurate 'on/off' charts in the busy hospital environment. At present there is no document available which is considered ideal for hospital use in all situations. However, this may in part be due to lack of time for completion, or poor understanding, rather than a criticism of current documents. When possible the patient should be asked to complete a chart or diary. Self-administration, both for completing diaries and giving medications, is probably the most effective method in terms of accuracy, and can give the patient a feeling of control. However, it is not always practical or appropriate, and the assessment process of an inpatient should include consideration of their ability to self-administer.

Key points

Assessments in the complex stage should include:

- Building a comprehensive picture of all the symptoms being experienced and highlight recent changes
- Normal coping strategies used to overcome these problems

- Identifying what is the worst problem at present and expectation and commitment to treatment
- Educational needs of the patient and their family
- The role of intercurrent health problems and the effects on PD control
- Suitability for self-administration

Palliative stage

Between 80% and 90% of people with PD will remain at home throughout their lives with most of their care provided by their families (Carter et al 1998). In the palliative stage the paradigm suggests the aim of treatment is to relieve symptoms and distress, maintain dignity and function and avoid treatment-related side effects. Assessments must therefore consider whether problems are symptoms or side effects and determine levels of discomfort and disability. For most this will lead to a gradual reduction of medications, retaining enough to maintain comfort and maximum possible function. As PD treatments are gradually reduced it may be necessary to introduce other drugs, such as analgesics, to maintain comfort and relieve distress.

The needs of the carer and family should also be reviewed and the Caregiver Strain Index (Robinson 1983) can be a useful tool. Both physical and psychological problems should be considered, as many carers say they can manage quite a high level of physical care but struggle with their own, and their relatives', psychological problems. Miller et al (1996) found that 40% of carers showed signs of strain and suggested that many admissions to long-term care occur because of breakdown of the carer's health as opposed to deterioration in the health of the PD patient.

Key points

Assessment in the palliative stage should include:

- Symptoms versus side effects
- Levels of discomfort and disability
- Needs of the family
- Long-term care needs

Common difficulties in assessing PD

In addition to the limitations of available assessment tools, other difficulties commonly occur when conducting a PD assessment, in particular 'on/off' fluctuations, communication difficulties and cognitive and psychiatric problems. Each of these will be explored in more detail although other chapters may cover the subject more fully and can be used for further reference.

'On' and 'off' fluctuations

'On' and 'off' fluctuations may be so severe that Koller (1999) suggests it can be like assessing two different people, one who is dysfunctional in the 'off' state and one who is functional in the 'on' state. An assessment of the true picture should therefore include both states. This can be difficult to achieve in practice, but it can be undertaken by the PDNS, where available, as they have sufficient flexibility in their role to see patients at different times of the day and in different settings. During an 'off' state many patients will be unable to speak coherently, sit upright or maintain eye contact; they may experience breathlessness, limb dysthaesia, abdominal pain, sweating, nausea, urinary urgency and frequency, anxiety, panic and depression. These problems can make assessment very difficult, and even experienced professionals express difficulty in making objective assessments during severe 'off' states.

While 'on', many patients will not wish to discuss their 'off' states, as they prefer to get on with life again and make the most of being mobile. In addition to wanting to forget 'bad times', many patients and carers have difficulty finding language to describe their experiences accurately. Awenat (1999) solved some of these problems by using video recordings for assessment. The equipment was initially used in outpatient clinics and hospital wards, and later lent to carers to record 'on' and 'off' states at home. Video recordings are now widely used to enhance patient assessments and to evaluate response to treatment.

To develop the assessment picture further it is useful to ask about a normal day; discussing an 'average' day is, perhaps, a slight misnomer as patients of all ages, and at all stages of the disease, experience good and bad days. If variable patterns and fluctuations are a concern, asking patients to complete a diary can be very useful. Several types of diaries are available, most needing completion at frequent intervals highlighting symptoms, food intake and medications. Many patients and carers enjoy keeping these records and understand their value in making decisions about treatment. When a patient or carer has taken time to complete a diary it should be viewed carefully, as it is common to hear the complaint that hours were spent on completing the diary yet the doctor gave it only a cursory glance.

Communication problems

Studies by Oxtoby (1982) found that almost 50% of people with PD had some problems with speech, although Marks et al (2001) suggests that most ignore or deny this until it markedly interferes with everyday life. Particular problems seen are low volume, reduced intonation, monotonous tone, stuttering, breathy or whispery speech, word blocking, disrupted sequencing, repetition, poor respiratory control with hurried or mumbled speech and poor auditory comprehension. These difficulties can make the assessment process very difficult, particularly if the listener has poor hearing or the assessment is conducted in a noisy environment.

Poor dentition and ill-fitting dentures may also affect the ability to speak coherently, and a dental health assessment should be included. Bradykinesia and rigidity can contribute to poor dental hygiene and tremor and dyskinesia can hamper dental treatments. Xerostomia, or dry mouth, and drooling are other common problems which cause poor dental hygiene, and discomfort and social embarrassment may render the patient unwilling or unable to talk for long periods.

Altered postures, poor body image, fixed facies, or mask-like expression may affect the normal non-verbal aspects of communication and may make a comprehensive assessment difficult to achieve, especially when combined with fatigue and poor motivation. Bradyphrenia, or slowness of thought, may cause delay in processing an answer to a question and extra time should be allowed for the patient to answer in order to avoid their being labelled confused or uninterested.

A recent study (Findley et al 2000) found that 75% of people with PD reported difficulty in writing, due to microphagia or tremor. When choosing an assessment tool for self-completion this should therefore be considered, as patients may be able to tick boxes, or write one or two words, but not be able to write sentences to give more qualitative information.

Psychiatric and psychological problems

It is not the remit of this chapter to discuss, in detail, the psychological and psychiatric problems that can occur with PD but there are some specific problems which may affect the assessment process. These include cognitive impairment, dementia, depression, anxiety and psychosis (Hindle 2001).

Types of psychological and psychiatric problems

Cognitive impairment

Cognitive impairment in PD is thought particularly to affect the ability to complete complex psychomotor tasks and the processes involved in learning, perception, intuition and reasoning (Hodges 1994). These changes make people with PD more likely to act reactively rather than predictively and cause difficulty with planning, memory and sequencing (Hindle 2001). This is particularly noticeable when they try to perform more than one task at a time. When conducting assessments it is better to ask questions when the person is seated, or at rest, rather than when walking or completing a motor activity.

Dementia

The overall incidence of dementia with PD is thought to be about 20% but it is more frequently seen in elderly patients (Clarke 2001). Typical manifestations are poor short-term memory, fluctuating confusion and visual hallucinations. Dementia associated with PD is thought to be the result of a spectrum of disorders, which need very careful assessment. This will be most effectively managed by psychiatric and physical teams working together (Hindle 2001). Assessments should include cognition, mental capacity, mood and psychosis, as well as motor and social function.

Depression

Depression in PD is common, around 64% in a recent study, but recognition and treatment is often poor (Meara 1999). Many of the symptoms of depression and PD are similar and depression in PD is often slightly different from a normal clinical depression and perhaps less severe (Clarke 2001). It is unclear whether the cause of depression in PD is altered biology or the social effects of having a chronic neurological disorder, but an assessment of mood should be made at all stages, as antidepressant therapy can be very effective (Clarke 2001).

Anxiety

Symptoms of anxiety are also very common in many people with PD, and may be related to depression, cognitive changes, 'off' states or change in social circumstances (Hindle 2001). Raised anxiety levels can lead to an apparent exacerbation of PD symptoms, particularly tremor; the patient should therefore be made to feel as comfortable as possible when being assessed.

Psychosis

The spectrum of psychosis in PD can vary widely from vivid dreams and occasional nightmares through to illusions, paranoid delusions and visual hallucinations. The most common causes are underlying Lewy body dementia and side effects of medication (Clarke 2001). Some people live happily with a mild degree of psychosis but, in most cases, prompt assessment and action is required. Studies by Goetz and Stebbins (1995) found that the development of hallucinations and delusions with PD were the strongest predictors of pending need for transfer to long-term care and the quality and breadth of assessment at this time was paramount.

Key points

- The aim of intervention should be to improve or maintain the patient's quality of life. Priority should be given to resolving the difficulties that are of most concern to patients and carers themselves
- Traditional approaches to treating PD focus on managing motor function, but current approaches recognize the additional importance of cognitive and emotional changes and how these affect the wider aspects of patients' lives
- A person with PD is likely to experience a wide spectrum of problems and the most effective assessments are those undertaken from a multi-professional perspective
- No comprehensive assessment tool is currently available, but patient problems and treatment options can be identified by using existing tools in conjunction with the pathway approach to underpin knowledge of the likely disease progression

References

Awenat Y (1999) The use of video recording in the assessment and management of Parkinson's disease. In: R Percival and P Hobson (eds.) Parkinson's Disease: Studies in Psychological and Social Care. London: BPS pp. 270–273.

Canter C J, De la Torre R and Mier M A (1992) Northwestern University Disability Scales. In: D T Wade (ed.) Measurement in Neurological Rehabilitation. New York: Oxford University Press pp. 325–327.

Carter JH, Stewart BJ and Archbold PG (1998) Living with a person who has Parkinson's disease: the spouse's perspective by stage of disease. Movement Disorders 13: 20–28.

Clarke C (2001) Parkinson's Disease in Practice. London: Royal Society of Medicine.

Ellgring H, Seiler S, Perleth B, Frings W, Gasser T and Oertel W (1993) Psychosocial aspects of Parkinson's disease. Neurology 43(Suppl 6): S41–44.

Fahn S and Elton R L (1987) Unified Parkinson's Disease Rating Scale. In: Fahn S, Marsden C D, Calne D B and Goldstein M (eds) Recent Developments in Parkinson's Disease, volume 2. New York: Macmillan pp. 153–163.

Findley L, Pugner K, Holmes J, Maker M and MacMahon D (2000) The impact of Parkinson's disease on quality of life: results of a research survey in the UK. Movement Disorders 15 (9 Suppl 3): 179.

Fitzpatrick R and Alonso J (1999) Quality of life in health care: concepts and components. In: P Martin and W Koller (eds.) Quality of Life in Parkinson's Disease. Barcelona: Masson pp. 1–16.

Goetz C G and Stebbins G T (1995) Mortality and hallucinations in nursing home patients with advanced Parkinson's. Neurology 45: 669–671.

Hindle J (2001) Neuropsychiatry. In: J Playfer and J Hindle (eds.) Parkinson's Disease in the Older Patient. London: Arnold pp. 106–133.

Hodges J R (1994) Cognitive Assessment for Clinicians. Oxford: Oxford University Press.

Hoehn M M and Yahr M D (1967) Parkinsonism: onset, progression and mortality. Neurology 17: 427–442.
Jenkinson C, Peto V, Fitzpatrick R, Greenhall R and Hyman N (1995) Self–reported functioning and well–being in patients with Parkinson's disease: comparison of the Short-form Health Survey (SF-36) and the Parkinson's Disease Questionnaire (PDQ-39). Age and Ageing 24: 505–509.
Koller W (1999) Drug treatment for Parkinson's disease: impact on the patient's quality of life. In: P Martin and W Koller (eds.) Quality of Life in Parkinson's Disease. Barcelona: Masson pp. 79–92.
Koplas P A, Gans H B and Wisely M P (1999) Quality of life and Parkinson's disease. Journal of Gerontology 54: 197–202.
Lincoln N and Radford K (1999) Driving and Parkinson's disease. In: R Percival and P Hobson (eds.) Parkinson's Disease: Studies in Psychological and Social Care. London: BPS pp. 274–283.
Llach X and Martin P (1999) Quality of life measurement: interest and applications. In: P Martin and W Koller (eds.) Quality of Life in Parkinson's Disease. Barcelona: Masson pp. 17–36.
MacMahon D and Thomas S (1998) Practical approach to quality of life in Parkinson's disease. Journal of Neurology 245(Suppl 1): S19–22.
MacMahon D (2001) Organization of services, concepts of management and health economics. In: J Playfer and J Hindle (eds.) Parkinson's Disease in the Older Patient. London: Arnold pp. 215–249.
Marks L, Hyland K M and Fiske J (2001) Oral considerations: communication and swallowing problems, diet and oral care. In: J Playfer and J Hindle (eds.) Parkinson's Disease in the Older Patient. London: Arnold pp. 134–164.
Meara R J, Mitchelmore E and Hobson J P (1999) Use of the GDS-15 geriatric depression scale as a screening instrument for depressive symptomatology in patients with Parkinson's disease and their carers in the community. Age and Ageing 28: 35–38.
Meara R J (2001) Assessment. In: J Playfer and J Hindle (eds.) Parkinson's Disease in the Older Patient. London: Arnold pp. 77–88.
Miller E, Berrios G E and Politynska B E (1996) Caring for someone with Parkinson's disease: factors that contribute to distress. International Journal of Geriatric Psychiatry 11: 263–268.
Morgan E and Moran M (2001) The Parkinson's disease nurse specialist. In: J Playfer and J Hindle (eds.) Parkinson's Disease in the Older Patient. London: Arnold pp. 273–282.
Oxtoby M (1982) Parkinson's Disease Patients and their Social Needs. London: PDS.
Parkinson J (1817) An Essay on the Shaking Palsy. London: Macmillan and PDS.
Robinson B C (1983) Validation of a Caregiver Strain Index. Journal of Gerontology 46: 507–512.
Struck A E, Siu A L, Wieland G D, Adams J and Rubenstein L Z (1993) Comprehensive geriatric assessment: a meta-analysis of controlled trials. Lancet 342: 1032–1036.
Webster D D (1968) Critical analyses of the disability in Parkinson's disease. Modern Treatment 5: 257–282.

CHAPTER TWELVE

Caring for a person with progressive supranuclear palsy

TESS ASTBURY AND MAGGIE ROSE

Clinical characteristics of progressive supranuclear palsy

Progressive supranuclear palsy (PSP) is a chronic neurodegenerative disease which affects the brain stem and basal ganglia. The clinical features of PSP are characterized by disturbance of balance, typically with falling backwards, impairment of mobility, disordered downward gaze and progressive disorder of speech and swallowing.

In the 1950s Dr Clifford Richardson studied a group of patients who had an unusual collection of neurological symptoms, including supranuclear ophthalmoplegia, dystonia, rigidity of the limbs, pseudobulbar palsy and dementia. He invited Dr John Steele and Dr Jerzy Olszewski to study the pathological changes, and they published the first clear description of PSP (Steele et al 1964). The following year, Barbeau (1965) proposed calling the disease Steele–Richardson–Olszewski syndrome, a name which some people still use today.

The cause of PSP is unknown. The incidence is approximately the same in men and women (Burn and Lees 2002). The usual age of onset is between the fifth and seventh decade though occasionally it is seen in much younger patients. The prognosis for people with PSP is poor. Life expectancy on average is around 5–7 years from onset of symptoms (Santacruz et al 1998) but some individuals may survive much longer.

A recent study in the north of England indicated a prevalence figure for PSP of 6.5/100,000 but it is suspected that the true number may be higher as a result of misdiagnosis or cases not being identified (Nath et al 2001). In one study by the Parkinson's Disease Society Brain Bank, 6% of patients dying with a clinical diagnosis of Parkinson's disease (PD) in fact had PSP at autopsy (Hughes et al 1992).

Pathology of PSP

Characteristically there are destructive changes in the basal ganglia and brain stem, with large numbers of neurofibrillary tangles, neurophil threads and tufted astrocytes. These distinctive histopathological inclusions are made up of insoluble aggregates of tau protein (Hauw et al 1994).

Diagnosis of PSP

The diagnosis is made on the presenting clinical picture. The diagnosis of PSP may be difficult as the early symptoms of the illness are often similar to those seen in PD and therefore a patient may have symptoms of PSP for some years before a diagnosis is reached. PSP has often been referred to as a 'Parkinson's plus' syndrome.

There are no universally accepted diagnostic tests for PSP although, in some centres, MRI brain scans may be requested. Specialized MRI scanning techniques are being developed which may assist more accurate diagnosis. These include measurement of the midbrain diameter on routine MRI (Warmuth-Metz et al 2001) and the use of a scoring system of recognizable MRI pointers (cortical atrophy, midbrain atrophy and third ventricle enlargement) in differentiating PSP from PD (Yekhlef et al 2003).

Early and accurate diagnosis, wherever possible, should be given in a sympathetic and understanding manner. The diagnosis is often distressing for both the patient and the carer, and support at the time of diagnosis can make a considerable difference. Appropriate information should be made available to the patient and family. If a Nurse Specialist is not on hand to give support, details of the PSP Association should be made available so that the family has access to accurate information about symptomatic treatment and support.

Management of PSP

With any long-term illness, such as PSP, the general practitioner (GP) may be best placed to coordinate care as they may know the patient and family well, and will be the first point of contact throughout the patient's time at home. The GP will also know what resources are available locally. The patient may only see their neurologist infrequently in a hospital outpatient department, sometimes many miles from home.

In best practice, when a diagnosis of possible or probable PSP is given, the neurologist should advise the GP to involve the multidisciplinary team. This should include:

- The Nurse Specialist (either the PSP nurse, the PD nurse or a neurology nurse with an interest in PSP)
- The speech and language therapist (SALT)
- The occupational therapist (OT)
- The physiotherapist

Good communication between the members of the multidisciplinary team and the patient and carers is essential for good quality care. A care plan should be drawn up by Social Services, pulling all the support services together. The patient should be allocated a care manager who can coordinate appropriate levels of support at home. Social Services may also be able to advise on claiming benefits such as Housing Benefit, Attendance Allowance or Disability Living Allowance. Depending on the stage of the illness, the district nurse, continence adviser and dietician may also become involved.

It is important for the family to be made aware of the potential danger of a person with PSP driving. Not only is it likely that reaction time will be slower, but there is also a tendency to veer to one side of the road. A driver has a legal obligation to inform the Driver and Vehicle Licensing Authority (DVLA) of any disability that they know they have. The medical officers at the DVLA will make enquiries about the medical condition and will decide whether a patient may continue to hold a licence. Although this may prove a difficult subject to raise, it is essential for the safety of all involved that the topic is not avoided.

Drug management of PSP

There is no specific drug therapy recommended for PSP but patients are often given a trial of levodopa or amantadine. These drugs occasionally have a mild beneficial effect in the early stages of the disease. Antiparkinsonian drugs may help with balance problems and stiffness, although their benefit is usually short-lived, and long-term use is usually avoided because of the side effects. Some neurologists will prescribe a tricyclic antidepressant such as amitriptyline. These drugs can help to lift mood but also have the added benefit of drying secretions due to the antimuscarinic (anticholinergic) side effect of this class of drug (discussed more fully in Chapter 9).

Management of the main symptoms of PSP

Balance problems

In PSP falling is common, and patients often fall backwards without warning. One of the strongest arguments for informing a family of the diagnosis of PSP, if it is suspected, is to make them aware of the potential hazard of falling backwards, especially on stairs. Falls are often initiated by turning too quickly or by making sudden movements. The additional difficulties of alteration to the downward gaze and an unsteady gait may increase the risk of falls. General information about safe mobilization is given in Table 12.1.

Table 12.1 General information to promote safe mobilization in PSP

- People with PSP should not be hurried when mobilizing
- Avoid low furniture, such as coffee tables, and loose rugs which can become hazardous
- The occupational therapist should visit and advise on grab rails, ramps and alterations to the home wherever appropriate
- The physiotherapist should be involved to advise on an exercise programme
- The physiotherapist may also advise on the use of wheeled frames and wheelchairs
- Lightweight zimmer frames are generally not suitable for patients with PSP as the motion of lifting the frame forwards can be enough to cause loss of balance
- Use of a more substantial wheeled frame, possibly weighted at the front, is a much safer option
- Most patients with PSP ultimately require a wheelchair because of immobility and falls. This should be comfortable and should provide adequate pressure relief and support
- In the more advanced stages of the illness, hoists may be required to assist in transfers
- A specially designed helmet, which can be provided by the surgical appliance department at the local hospital, may avoid serious head injury and unnecessary and traumatic trips to casualty

Visual problems

Although visual acuity itself is unaffected by PSP, patients with PSP lose the ability to move their eyes fully up and (more importantly) down. Characteristically, this inability to look down is accompanied by extension of the head and a fixed wide-eyed stare (Morris et al 1999). On examination, a full range of vertical eye movements can be elicited by the doll's eye manoeuvre (passively moving the patient's head up and down).

There may be a variety of other visual disorders in PSP, the most common being double vision. This occurs due to loss of eye convergence (where the eye muscles pull each eye inwards to focus on an near object). The inability to look down, coupled with possible double vision and slowed side-to-side movements, means that many patients are not able to read and find difficulty eating. Visual problems may increase the risk of falls, impair mobility and cause difficulty with communication.

Movements of the eyelids are also affected. The frequency of blinking may be slowed, leading to drying of the eyes and irritation or conjunctivitis. Blepharospasm (spasm in the eyelid muscles) is common and causes difficulty with eyelid opening. Not all people with PSP experience all the visual problems, and they can be reassured that they will not lose their sight totally, but almost all patients complain of some alteration to their vision. General advice on visual problems is given in Table 12.2.

Table 12.2 General advice on visual problems

- Place items such as call buzzers, food and drinks, and television control within the patient's field of vision
- Eye drops can be used to assist in moistening dry eyes
- Changing prescription for lenses is not likely to be of any benefit
- Prisms may be helpful to assist reading
- Different corrections may be required for different activities, e.g. reading or watching television
- Lid crutches (stiff wires which can gently hold the lids open) can be attached to spectacles
- Injections of botulinum toxin may be given into the eyelid to help treat blepharospasm in severe cases
- Consider referral to an ophthalmologist for an assessment. They may consider registering the patient as blind, thus enabling 'talking books' and 'talking newspapers' to be obtained free of charge. The patient may also be entitled to benefits such as reduced council tax, television licence and travel costs

Swallowing problems

Patients with PSP invariably develop problems with swallowing. This causes great distress and is potentially dangerous as there is an increased risk of choking and aspiration. Involvement with the SALT is extremely important and the patient should be referred as soon as the diagnosis has been made. An early assessment is always beneficial and reassures both the patient and the carer. If dysphagia is present then safe swallowing techniques can be taught and advice on the texture of food offered. General advice regarding safe swallowing is given in Table 12.3.

Table 12.3 General advice regarding safe swallowing

- Early referral to SALT is essential
- Patients should not be rushed when eating
- Good posture whilst eating is important, sitting up and slightly forwards
- Solid food should be softened
- Liquid drinks should be thickened using a preparation such as 'Thick and Easy'
- Patient should be referred to a dietician for advice on energy intake
- Monitor food and fluid intake
- Monitor weight. People with PSP are vulnerable to malnutrition and dehydration and need to be monitored closely

A videofluoroscopy examination may be useful to assess the degree of reduction to the swallowing reflex. Where there is a recurring danger of aspiration pneumonia, or if feeding is becoming stressful or prolonged and the swallow difficult to initiate, the SALT together with the neurologist, and the patient and their family, may wish to discuss the possibility of feeding via a percutaneous endoscopic gastrostomy (PEG). It is often better to raise the issue of alternative feeding early in the illness when the patient's levels of comprehension and communication are better. Understandably, some families find this a difficult subject to approach but it is better to discuss these issues in a planned way rather than when an emergency situation has arisen.

In any condition when dysphagia is expected to be present for more than a few weeks, the use of a gastrostomy tube is preferable to nasogastric intubation (Pennington 2002). Nasogastric tubes are usually poorly tolerated and may make the patient agitated; many patients will pull the tube out. In addition, the volume of feed delivered by this route is often inadequate. Nasogastric tubes may be associated with complications such as nasopharyngitis, oesophagitis and epistaxis and they do not fully protect against aspiration. Gastrostomy tube feeding is more likely to deliver the appropriate daily nutrition (Park et al 1992).

Speech problems

As PSP progresses, patients often develop dysarthria (difficulty with the articulation of speech). The voice often becomes strained and husky or may become so quiet that it is impossible to discern what is being said. Some people become stuck on words and repeat the same thing over and over again (perseverance). Often there is a problem with initiating speech even though the person knows what they want to say. There are a few simple things which may help with communication and these are listed in Table 12.4.

Table 12.4 Practical advice to promote effective communication

- Avoid excess background noise
- Try to be at the same level and maintain eye contact
- Don't rush the patient – wait for a response
- The strength of the voice usually fluctuates during the day, so it is helpful to utilize the 'good' times
- The SALT may be able to give vocal exercises
- Communication aids can be provided and may be of some benefit providing there is good hand/eye coordination. Electronic aids, such as Lightwriters, may be helpful for a short while but, in practice, more simple gadgets such as alphabet boards or picture boards may be of more use
- Microphones or speech amplifiers will help to amplify a quiet voice, and plug-in loudspeakers are available for use with the telephone
- A communication booklet is helpful if communication problems are severe. This could contain details about the patient, such as likes and dislikes, and key phrases as well as some general information about the patient. This allows visiting carers to refer to the book and learn something about the patient to make everyday 'conversation' less strained

Many people with PSP suffer the distressing and embarrassing symptom of drooling saliva. This is not because they make excessive amounts of saliva but because they have reduced swallowing, allowing the saliva to collect in the mouth and trickle out (Bakheit 2001.) Sometimes prescribing the antidepressant drug amitriptyline, to utilize the side effect of drying secretions, is enough to control this symptom. In more severe cases hyoscine tablets or scopolamine patches may be successful in treating the symptoms (Talmi et al 1990). Occasionally suction may be used to help clear the back of the mouth.

Behavioural change

In the early stages of the illness there are often subtle changes in behaviour or personality which may include concentration lapses and depression. Although intellect may remain intact, there may be problems with short-term memory, understanding, reason, irritability or general apathy. Neuropsychiatric symptoms are common in basal ganglia disorders such as PSP and PD but there appear to be differences in the types of symptoms which occur in these two diseases. Patients with PSP tend to show significantly more apathy and disinhibition whereas patients with PD have a higher frequency of hallucinations, delusions and depression (Aarsland et al 2001). The cognitive deficit in PSP is widespread and independent of depression. There is also thought to be an association between the severity of the eye movement disorder and deficits in attention (Esmonde et al 1996).

Carers often talk about 'living with a stranger'. A typical example to illustrate this lack of understanding would be the case of a patient who is prone to falling, whose wife asks him to sit still while she briefly leaves the room. He fails to understand the instruction or the implication of not obeying it. The minute her back is turned he gets up, overbalances and crashes to the floor. Understanding these cognitive changes may help the carer to cope.

Depression

Depression commonly occurs in PSP and often may not be recognized. Depression is a common co-morbidity of many chronic illnesses that can exacerbate the effects of the medical condition and be an independent source of suffering and disability (Gaynes et al 2002). Increasingly, neurologists prescribe antidepressant medication for patients with PSP. These drugs not only help to elevate mood but also in some people have the additional benefit of briefly improving the symptoms of balance and speech.

Pain in PSP

PSP in itself does not give rise to pain, but patients can experience symptomatic pain as the illness progresses. Patients often experience pain or discomfort in the neck as a result of restricted movement and stiffness. This pain may be localized or referred, radiating down into the shoulders or upwards causing headache. The application of warmth, massage or analgesia may be of some benefit. Sometimes muscle-relaxing drugs are prescribed, but without much success, and injections of botulinum toxin into the neck muscle may be tried.

PSP patients may experience cramp-like pain in the limbs. Simple measures such as passive and active exercises can be helpful. The application of heat or massage, or use of simple analgesics, may be beneficial. It is worth bearing in mind that a PSP patient's pain may be due to another medical condition that may warrant investigation.

Urinary and bowel problems

As the disease progresses and the patient becomes increasingly immobile, problems such as constipation and urinary dysfunction may occur. Constipation is managed in the early stages by making changes to the diet to include adequate fruit and roughage and sufficient fluid intake. This may become less easy as swallowing becomes compromised, and the use of laxatives may be required. In the later stages, suppositories or enemas may be necessary to stimulate the bowels to open.

With increasing weakness and difficulty with mobility, bladder management often becomes more difficult. Patients need more help to get to the toilet. Some patients experience difficulty initiating the flow of urine, and some need to be up frequently at night. This can be exhausting for the carer. Practical advice to promote urinary continence is illustrated in Table 12.5.

Table 12.5 Practical advice to promote urinary continence

- Consider whether there may be a urinary infection
- Encourage a good fluid intake
- Refer patients to the local continence advice nurse for individual assessment of the urinary dysfunction
- Various aids are available, such as bottles and commodes, pads and catheters
- Discuss with both the patient and the carer about the equipment of choice
- Intermittent catheterization works well for some people and allows total emptying of the bladder
- Other patients may choose to have a permanent catheter

Complementary therapies in PSP

Because of the lack of conventional treatments for PSP many patients try alternative therapies. These include homeopathic and herbal remedies, acupuncture and reflexology. Although none of these have been shown to be universally helpful, some people do gain some relief. This, of course, may be due at least in part to the placebo effect. People with PSP should always seek help from accredited therapists and talk to their GP about any alternative treatments they may be considering.

Palliative care in PSP

PSP is an immensely individual illness but, in all cases, as the condition progresses so the role of the carer increases. With developing immobility comes increased stiffness, difficulty with movement, possible contractures causing pain and susceptibility to pressure sores. By this stage communication may be extremely difficult, adding to the patient's frustration. Urinary tract infections and incontinence are both common. Respiratory tract infections increase as the cough reflex becomes weakened and the danger of aspirating food becomes more real. This can prove fatal, if it is unnoticed and treatment is delayed, so any signs of a chest infection should warrant an early referral to the GP allowing antibiotics to be prescribed.

Patients with advanced PSP should be referred to the palliative care team. These teams are better known for their work with terminally ill cancer patients, but are increasingly becoming involved with the care of patients with degenerative neurological conditions, such as motor neurone disease and PSP (neuro-palliative care). The role of the palliative care team is to try to relieve symptoms and anxiety for the patient, to support the family and carer and to work closely with anyone else involved in the care of the patient, such as therapists, nurses or doctors. Adequate support for the carer, both practical and emotional, is extremely important. Provision of short-term respite care or day care, in either a nursing home or a hospice, may give the carer a much-needed break and enable care at home to continue. The palliative care philosophy can help direct the patient's hope from cure to a palliative goal (Sjostrom et al 2002).

At this stage of the illness the patient's quality of life must always be considered, with the emphasis on symptom control. Analgesia should be given where appropriate. Muscle relaxant drugs or injections of botulinum toxin can be administered if necessary. In the final stages of the illness, invasive, intensive medical treatment, such as cardiopulmonary resuscitation or mechanical ventilation, would not normally be considered appropriate, but should always be discussed on an individual basis.

The role of the PSP Association and the PSP Nurse Specialist

The PSP Association provides information and support to help raise awareness of the condition. The Association is a fund-raising charity which works to support research into PSP. The revelation that the actor and musician Dudley Moore had PSP helped increase the awareness of the illness and in some cases has helped families of sufferers feel less isolated. The Association promotes educational meetings for professionals, and organizes support groups for patients and their carers. The Association employs two PSP Nurse Specialists.

In the early days after diagnosis, the specialist nurse is able to supply families with information about the illness as well as reassuring them about the support available, both in the community through the multidisciplinary team, and over the telephone.

The main role of the PSP Nurse Specialists is to run a telephone helpline to give patients and carers advice, information and support whenever they need it. Each nurse attends the regular support group meetings in their area. These meetings are held in various locations throughout the country. The meetings enable carers (and occasionally patients) to come together to share experiences, to exchange telephone numbers, to hear what is happening with PSP in the field of research (drug trials, etc.), and, above all, to gain mutual support. These meetings also allow the Nurse Specialists a chance to get to know the carers they speak to on the telephone.

The Nurse Specialists also fulfil an important role in education, giving talks to GPs, SALTs, other specialist nurses, or care workers at residential or nursing homes. They attend study days on associated neurological conditions, both to increase their own knowledge and to network with fellow professionals. However, their main role is to support people with PSP and to help in any way that can improve the quality of life and alleviate the burden of the carer.

Key points

- PSP is a progressive neurodegenerative disease
- There is no known cure
- Life expectancy is 5–7 years from onset although some patients survive much longer
- Prevalence is estimated at 6.5 per 100,000 of population
- The main symptoms of PSP are:
  - Balance disturbance with falls, especially falling backwards
  - Visual problems, especially problems with downward gaze
  - Progressive problems with mobility
  - Speech and swallowing difficulties
  - Personality change
- The PSP Association offers information and support for patients and carers

PSP Association details

The PSP Association (The Progressive Supranuclear Palsy (PSP Europe) Association), The Old Rectory, Wappenham, Towcester NN12 8SQ.
Tel 01327 860299/342 Tel/Fax 01327 861007/113
E-mail psp.eur@virgin.net
Website www.pspeur.org

Helplines:
Maggie Rose RGN, RSCN (North) Tel 01939 270889
Tess Astbury RGN (South) Tel 01604 844825

References

Aarsland D, Litvan I and Larsen J P (2001) Neuropsychiatric symptoms of patients with progressive supranuclear palsy and Parkinson's disease. Journal of Neuropsychiatry and Clinical Neuroscience 13(1): 42–49.

Bakheit A M O (2001) Management of neurogenic dysphagia. Postgraduate Medical Journal 77(913): 694–699.

Barbeau A (1965) Degenerescence plurisystematisée du nevraxe. L'Union Medicale du Canada 94(6): 715–718.

Burn D J and Lees A J (2002) Progressive supranuclear palsy: where are we now? Lancet Neurology 1(6): 359–369.

Esmonde T, Giles E, Gibson M and Hodges J R (1996) Neuropsychological performance, disease severity and depression in progressive supranuclear palsy. Journal of Neurology 243(9): 638–643.

Gaynes B N, Burns B J, Tweed D L and Erickson P (2002) Depression and health-related quality of life. Journal of Nervous and Mental Disease 190(12): 799–806.

Hauw J J, Daniel S E, Dickson D, Horoupain D S, Jellinger K, Lantos P L, McKee A, Tabaton M and Litvan I (1994) Preliminary NINDS neuropathological criteria for Steel–Richardson–Olszewski syndrome (progressive supranuclear palsy). Neurology 44(11): 2015–2019.

Hughes A J, Daniel S E, Kilford L and Lees A J (1992) Accuracy of clinical diagnosis of idiopathic Parkinson's disease: a clinicopathological study of 100 cases. Journal of Neurology, Neurosurgery and Psychiatry 55(3): 181–184.

Morris H R, Wood N W and Lees A J (1999) Progressive supranuclear palsy (Steele–Richardson–Olszewski disease). Postgraduate Medical Journal 888: 579–584.

Nath U, Ben–Sholomo Y, Thomson R G et al. (2001) The prevalance of progressive supranuclear palsy (Steele–Richardson–Olszewski syndrome) in the UK. Brain 124(7): 1438–1449.

Park R H R, Allison M C, Lag J et al (1992) Randomised comparison of percutaneous endoscopic gastrostomy and nasogastric tube feeding in patients with persisting neurological dysphagia. British Medical Journal 304(6839): 1406–1409.

Pennington C (2002) To PEG or not to PEG. Clinical Medicine 2(3): 250–255.

Santacruz P, Uttl B, Litvan I and Grafman J (1998) Progressive supranuclear palsy: a survey of the disease course. Neurology 50(6): 1637–1647.

Sjostrom A C, Holmberg B and Strang P (2002) Parkinson-plus patients – an unknown group with severe symptoms. Journal of Neuroscience Nursing 34(6): 314–319.

Steele J C, Richardson J C and Olszewski J (1964) Progressive supranuclear palsy. Archives of Neurology 10: 333–359.

Talmi Y P, Finkelstein Y and Zohar Y (1990) Reduction of salivary flow with transdermal scopolamine: a four year experience. Otolaryngology and Head and Neck Surgery 103(4): 615–618.

Warmuth-Metz M, Naumann M, Csoti I and Solymosi L (2001) Measurement of the midbrain diameter on routine magnetic resonance imaging: a simple and accurate method of differentiating between Parkinson disease and progressive supranuclear palsy. Archives of Neurology 58(7): 1076–1079.

Yekhlef F, Ballan G, Macia F, Delmer O, Sourgen C and Tison F (2003) Routine MRI for the differntial diagnosis of Parkinson's disease, MSA, PSP and CBD. Journal of Neural Transmission 110(2): 151–169.

CHAPTER THIRTEEN
Multiple system atrophy

CATHERINE BEST

Introduction

Multiple system atrophy (MSA) is not a well-recognized or well-understood disorder, despite the major disabling and life-shortening consequences for an individual with the diagnosis.

> Multiple system atrophy (MSA) is a sporadic progressive adult onset disorder characterized by a variable combination of autonomic features, parkinsonism and ataxia.
>
> Consensus Statement (1996)

This definition succeeds in neatly packing a wide and complex range of symptoms into a comprehensive order. If it were as easy to do in practice or when faced with a patient who may have movement difficulties or bladder problems, or is collapsing, there would be little need for this chapter. In reality, the variety of presenting features, the diagnostic difficulties, the sheer number of symptoms that a patient can experience and the variable rate of progression create a real challenge for nursing a patient with MSA.

This chapter seeks to explain what MSA actually is, to offer management strategies for many of the symptoms and to identify the key role for nurses in order to provide the best possible care for patients with MSA, their families and carers.

Confusion and consensus

In its 100-year history MSA has had a large number of names, creating confusion for patients and health professionals alike (Figure 13.1).

Since the 1900s each successive description, while adding to the neurological or pathological knowledge of MSA, also added to the number of

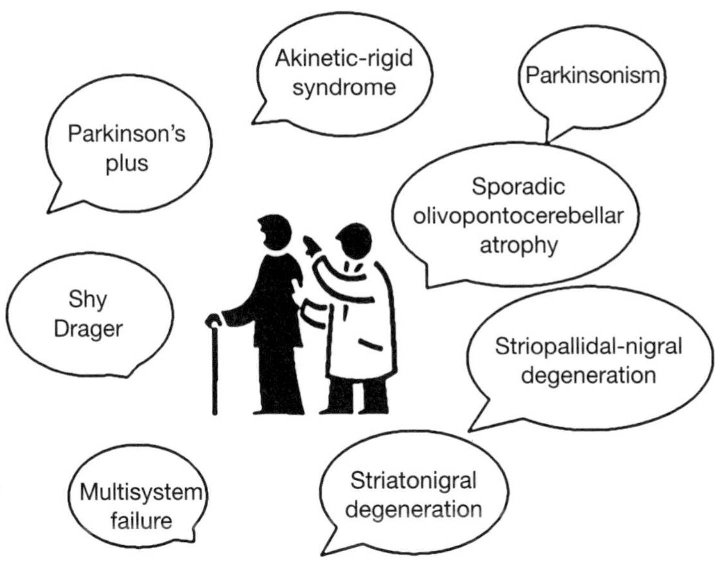

Figure 13.1 The many names of MSA.

names for the disease. Quinn (1989) sought to end this historical confusion (Table 13.1) by providing provisional diagnostic criteria.

Table 13.1 Significant historical MSA developments

Year	Author	Contribution to understanding MSA
1900	Dejerine and Thomas	Described olivopontocerebellar atrophy
1925	Bradbury and Eggleston	Case reports of postural hypotension
1960	Shy and Drager	Described autonomic features and neurology
1960	van der Eecker	Described striato-nigral degeneration
1969	Graham and Oppenheimer	Used the term multiple system atrophy
1989	Quinn	Putting everything together: 'The nature of the beast'

In order to understand the disease there needed to be clarity about what MSA is. It was also important to stop the use of the term to describe *any* collection of neurological symptoms that defied diagnosis. To this end, an international committee of doctors and scientists agreed by consensus upon a definition of MSA (Consensus Statement 1996).

The consensus committee working on the definition included physicians, neurologists and cardiologists all of who may be presented with patients with MSA. MSA does cross speciality boundaries, and subsequent initiatives (Table 13.2) reflect this.

Table 13.2 Recent MSA developments

1996	Definition consensus	Description of MSA
1999	Diagnosis consensus	Criteria for diagnosis (Gilman et al 1998)
1999	European MSA Study Group	Collaborative research network of clinical centres
2000	First clinical trial	Neuroprotection and Natural History in MSA and PSP (UK, France and Germany)

Initial presentation

Patients initially experience symptoms from one of three symptom groups: cerebellar, autonomic or parkinsonism. Over time further symptoms from the other groups develop and there is an overlap. Patients can be classified depending on their predominant group of symptoms (Figure 13.2).

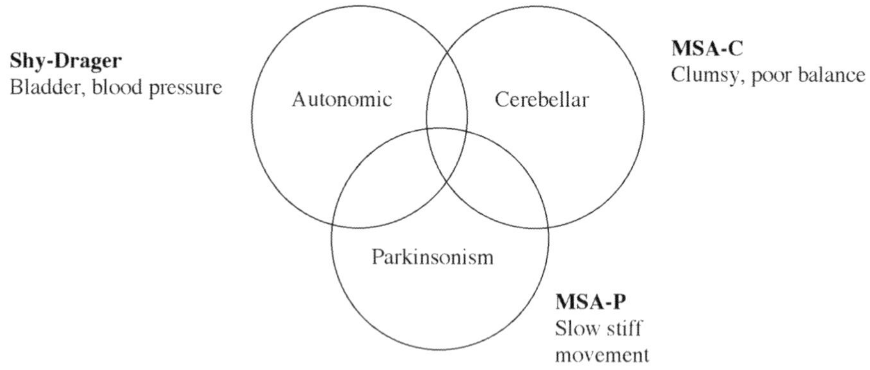

Figure 13.2 Symptom groups in MSA (adapted from Swan and Dupont 1999).

For men the first presenting sign is often erectile dysfunction (inability to achieve or sustain an erection) (Wenning et al 1999). Both men and women often have early bladder problems, urgency, frequency, incomplete bladder emptying or an inability to pass urine. These problems may go unreported if patients feel embarrassed or attribute them to ageing.

The development of movement problems is more likely to bring patients to seek advice from either a doctor or a physiotherapist. Early problems include stiffness and finding movement difficult or slower. Difficulty turning in bed or problems walking in crowded places are also common (Mathias and Bannister 2002). Handwriting may change, or patients can become clumsy or unsteady. Others may experience dizziness when standing up or may even faint.

It is difficult for patients to connect their diverse symptoms together, especially if they develop at different times. Initial referrals to different specialists may not make a connection between these early problems either.

These are general patterns of presentation and, like all generalizations, cannot reflect all individual patients, some of whom present with very specific problems, such as stridor or dysphagia. For nurses, getting as much information as possible from the patient and keeping an open mind, especially when working in specialist practice, are key skills needed to identify MSA.

Getting a diagnosis

The presenting symptoms of MSA mimic other disorders. In a survey of Sarah Matheson Trust members in 2000, 58% had a first diagnosis of PD. Of the other 42% very few obtained MSA as a first diagnosis; most were thought to have ataxia, autonomic failure or even depression. This is by no means a reflection of poor diagnostic skills but of the tricky nature of MSA.

These difficulties are a challenge for clinicians, but a real cause of frustration to patients. The tortuous route to diagnosis for patients may involve several different specialists, trials of drugs that are ineffective or even surgery that makes things worse, all with the anxiety of waiting times. Depending on how this journey is managed, patients may feel disillusioned with health professionals by the time a diagnosis of MSA is made.

Quinn (1989) and Gilman et al (1998) suggest diagnostic criteria for MSA. They consist of combination of criteria for 'probable', 'possible' or 'definite diagnosis'. A definite diagnosis can only be made on postmortem examination of the brain. Both methods require considerable thought and are not easily used in clinical settings. A system of 'red flags' may be more useful. These are symptoms that raise awareness of the possibility of MSA (Table 13.3).

Table 13.3 'Red flags' (symptoms that raise awareness of the possibility of MSA)

Poor response to levodopa	Postural hypotension
Erectile dysfunction	Early bladder disturbance
Cold extremities	Early dysphonia, dysarthria or dysphagia
Inspiratory sighs	Respiratory stridor
Rapid progression, early use of wheelchair	

Studies from brain research centres show that diagnostic accuracy is increasing (Ansorge et al 2002), but this is not an indication that the diagnosis is occurring earlier in the disease. Currently a diagnosis is given after taking a thorough medical history, performing a neurological examination and eliminating other potential causes for the present symptoms. Tests that are usually performed include:

- MRI scans to detect structural changes to the brain. If changes are visible (and often they may not be) they can support an MSA diagnosis, but the absence of changes does not rule out MSA (Schrag et al 1998)
- Genetic screening to differentiate between sporadic ataxia and MSA
- Sphincter EMG to assesses the nerve supply to the bladder or bowel outlet, which is impaired in MSA. It can be useful to support a diagnosis of MSA although there is some debate about its use, depending on the range of measurements assessed
- Formal autonomic testing can determine the extent of cardiovascular autonomic dysfunction and differentiate between other causes of autonomic failure. Future autonomic investigation with cardiac scanning may be able to differentiate between MSA and PD

A diagnostic tool that is a reliable, non-invasive, easy to access and widely available remains a distant hope.

Neuropathology

Postmortem examination of the brain shows cell damage and loss, together with the presence of glial cytoplasmic inclusion bodies (Papp et al 1989). This occurs in areas involved in control of autonomic, cerebellar and movement functions (brain stem, cerebellum and basal ganglia). Glial cytoplasmic inclusion bodies are comet-shaped tangles of protein (alpha-synuclein) and are characteristic of MSA.

What else can happen?

As the disease progresses patients will not get every symptom listed below although they will experience many of them. Disease progression causes significant disabilities, reduces independence in all aspects of daily life and makes MSA very complex to manage.

Symptoms experienced during progression of MSA include:

- **Parkinsonism**
  Stiffness
  Difficulty in turning in bed

Writing becoming small or spidery
Difficulty initiating movement
Freezing
Antecollis
Falls

- **Cerebellar**
  Clumsy, dropping things
  Difficulty with fine coordination, e.g. fastening buttons
  Feeling unsteady in crowds
  Difficulty writing
  Slurred speech
  Unable to stand without support
  Falls

- **Autonomic**
  Bladder problems
  Erectile dysfunction
  Feeling dizzy or fainting
  Neck and shoulders pain
  Falls
  Constipation
  Cold hands and feet
  Inability to sweat
  Swallowing problems, choking (dysphagia)
  Snoring
  Inspiratory sighs
  Exaggerated startle response

- **Other problems**
  Weakness in arms and legs
  Heightened emotional response, laughing or crying
  Restless sleep, nightmares
  Weak, quiet, quivering voice

Progression and prognosis

MSA creates disabilities that greatly reduce independent function early in the disease (Muller et al 2000). The movement problems created by parkinsonism and ataxia are difficult to manage (Wenning and Braune 2001). Falls are 10 times more common than in patients with PD (Tison et al 2002) and the survival times once wheelchair-dependent are less than 1 year

(Muller et al 2000). Problems with swallowing also occur early (Muller et al 2001), which can cause dehydration or malnutrition; these increase patient discomfort, exacerbate other symptoms and can be life threatening.

MSA is a life-shortening disease. The mean life expectancy from the onset of symptoms is 6 years although rates vary from 1 to 24 years (Ben-Shlomo et al 1997). The most common cause of death is bronchopneumonia but sudden death in patients not in the most advanced stages can occur, often at night. The sudden death is thought to be the result of a significant autonomic cardiovascular or respiratory event.

Sarah Matheson Trust figures in 2001 suggest that the average time to get a diagnosis from initial symptoms to diagnosis is 2–5 years. This may leave the patient with very little time from diagnosis until death.

Prevalence

Just how common MSA actually is is difficult to determine; an underestimate in 1999 suggested by Schrag et al (2000) is 4.4 per 100,000. Compared to motor neurone disease at 7 per 100,000, this is no longer a rare disorder (The Neurological Alliance, 2003).

'Are there more people with MSA now?' is a question that patients often ask. Although it is difficult to say with certainty, the yearly increase of patients registered with the Sarah Matheson Trust is more likely to be because of greater awareness of the condition and improved access to neurological services.

Epidemiology

The mean age of onset is 54 years (Ben-Shlomo et al 1997) although symptoms can develop between the ages of 30 and 90. It occurs slightly more in men than women (1.3:1); the reason for this is not known. MSA occurs worldwide in white, African and Asian populations, and no genetic or familial links have yet been identified.

Management

First, and most important, the management of someone with MSA needs to be hopeful but realistic. Without hope, an individual becomes crushed by their situation and without realistic expectations for themselves, and they risk permanent dissatisfaction.

In the following section, specific problem management and an insight into the number of hospital and community services that may be involved in one person's care are considered. A truly interdisciplinary approach is needed to identify and coordinate the priorities of care. An interdisciplinary team needs to be able to:

- Be clear about the priorities. Given the volume of symptoms, it would be unrealistic to be able to manage them all. This is a degenerative condition so improving function may not be possible. Addressing the priorities for the patient with the abilities of the team is fundamental
- Communicate clearly in order to:
  - Understand the patient and their situation
  - Know who else is involved in the patient's care (there will be plenty!)
  - Understand what the patient has been told about diagnosis, treatment decisions like gastrostomy tube feeding, and dying
  - Understand what the patient feels about treatment options, taking part in research, dying and brain donation
  - Understand how family and carers feel
  - Keep up with any changes
- Provide the three Rs:
  - Reassessment as the condition changes; this may mean having to prioritize services, or not discharging patients who would have to go to the end of the queue with a new problem
  - Rapid response. Problems like infections that can cause massive deterioration need to be treated immediately
  - Respite care in the most appropriate setting. This could mean staying at home, using hospice facilities or a holiday cottage
- Offer carer support. For most patients a family member, usually a partner, is their primary carer. This is physically tiring, stressful and emotionally draining, and every professional who is involved should consider this

Management of specific problems

Movement

Drug treatment of movement problems may not be as effective in MSA as it is in PD, but it still has its place.

Poor response to levodopa

Levodopa may have a good effect initially, although this 'honeymoon effect' wanes over time (Wenning et al 1994). However, levodopa does seem to help reduce stiffness. Amantadine is also useful. Even if the patient appears not to obtain benefit from either of these therapies, care must be taken before stopping them however as alarming deterioration can occur (Quinn 1993). Levodopa may make some patients feel significantly worse. This is more likely to affect patients with autonomic features because of the hypotensive effect of levodopa. Levodopa can be given to patients with postural hypotension but may need to be given with medication to support blood pressure.

Ataxia

The deterioration in walking ability is best managed by use of aids that improve stability. These may only be useful for a limited time before a wheelchair becomes the most appropriate aid. Equipment to improve arm and hand coordination is limited, and the best help may be someone else to perform the task for the patient.

Tremor

It is unusual to see classic pill-rolling tremor. An intention tremor is more common and is associated with cerebellar problems. It can make tasks such as using cutlery or writing difficult. Built-up handles on pens may help initially. An occupational therapist can provide equipment such as a 'neater-eater' to minimize the tremor, but over time other people will be required to do these tasks.

Dystonia

This can affect limbs or face and neck. In patients with parkinsonian symptoms dystonia can respond well initially to levodopa, although peak-dose dyskinesia (writhing movements) may develop (Boesch et al 2002).

Antecollis

The position of the chin on the chest makes speech, swallowing and breathing more difficult. Chairs that 'tilt in space' are more useful than reclining chairs for positioning patients with antecollis. Neck collars or head straps can be useful for short periods but are uncomfortable for long-term use. They can be used to facilitate important discussions by restoring eye contact.

Unable to turn in bed

Coordinating all limbs, trunk and head to enable movement in bed is an early problem, which can be specifically worked at with a physiotherapist to refine the technique. An occupational therapist can provide bed rails or other equipment to help. Most people will depend on a partner or carer being taught to do this with sliding sheets. Community nurses can provide beds and mattresses to improve comfort. Controlled-release levodopa should also be considered.

Unable to get up the stairs

Stairs often create the biggest problems for patients. Using different floors with a stair lift or through-floor lift is an option if single-floor living is not possible. As with all home adaptations, how quickly they can be installed and at what expense must be considered against the practicalities of a short life expectancy.

Falls

Falls can occur for several reasons (Table 13.4). Detailed questioning is required to find the causes, and preventive action should be taken seriously because of the risk of injury.

Table 13.4 Causes of falls and appropriate action

	Cerebellar	**Parkinsonism**	**Autonomic**
Fall behaviour	Changing direction, turning around, losing balance	Sticky feet, freezing on the spot while upper body continues to move	Sudden falls sometimes preceded by dizziness. Associated after food, exertion or going to the toilet
Action	Re-educate to move or change direction slowly and gradually	Reassess use of PD medication	Assess lying and standing blood pressure. Provide postural hypotension advice and medication
Refer	Occupational therapist for education. Wheelchair clinic	Physiotherapist to improve postural stability	For autonomic testing. Occupational therapist for equipment such as perching stools

Postural hypotension

This symptom often occurs early in the disease. It merits attention as a symptom, if only for the fact that it can usually be well managed (Wenning and Braune 2001). It is sometimes called orthostatic hypotension.

Postural hypotension is a fall in blood pressure after 3 minutes of standing. The fall should be at least 20 mmHg systolic or 10 mmHg diastolic. The resulting reduced supply of blood to areas of the body gives rise to symptoms (Mathias 1998) (Table 13.5).

Table 13.5 Symptoms of postural hypotension according to area of poor blood supply.

Brain	Dizzy, lightheaded Changes in vision, greying tunnel or blurred vision Feeling vague or muddled
Muscles	Pain across shoulders and neck (coat-hanger pain) (Bleasdale-Barr and Mathias 1998) Pain in lower back or buttocks Angina-type pain Weakness
General	Fatigue

These are warning signs that herald losing consciousness (a blackout or faint), unless preventive measures are taken.

Why postural hypotension occurs in MSA

Blood pressure is regulated by nerves and hormones, which direct the flow and volume of blood circulating in the body. This maintains a blood supply to vital organs such as the brain and heart at all times, even when blood is needed for everyday activities like digesting food or performing exercise. In MSA the central control of autonomic nerves is affected and postural hypotension occurs as a result of the competing demands.

It is more likely to occur:

- When sitting up or standing up, when gravity acts by 'pulling blood towards the feet'
- In the morning when the normal diurnal pattern of blood pressure is low
- After activities that place greater blood supply demands, such as exercise, eating and digesting food, especially big meals or meals or drinks high in sugar
- Straining on the toilet to pass urine or faeces, which will cause a drop in blood pressure

It can also be made worse if the patient is dehydrated, during illness, e.g. a urinary infection, or by some medication.

Treatment

Treatment has a three-point approach: recognition, prevention and management.

Understanding the mechanism of postural hypotension and evaluating its effects, by asking the patient directly and by taking lying and standing blood pressure recordings, should reveal any evidence of postural hypotension.

Further evaluation of specific trigger factors such as food or exercise can be done with formal autonomic testing.

Treating other symptoms that affect blood pressure control such as reducing infections (managing bladder problems, having the flu jab) and preventing constipation (good fluid intake) will promote better blood pressure control.

There is a variety of non-pharmacological measures that will improve blood pressure control. These also have the advance of enabling the patient to retain choice in their treatment (Table 13.6).

Table 13.6 Non-pharmacological measures to improve blood pressure control

Things to do	Things to avoid
Raise head of bed up	Lying flat
Increase fluid and salt intake	Early morning activity
Change position slowly and in stages	Warm environments
Wiggle feet and ankles before moving	Standing still
Eat small meals and snacks	High-sugar foods and drinks
Plan activity throughout the day	Straining on the toilet

The medications most frequently used to support blood pressure include fludrocortisone, ephedrine, midodrine and desmopressin.

It is important to educate patients and carers to take evasive action at the onset of any of the symptoms of postural hypotension:

- Sit down or lie down, drink at least one glass of water
- Think about what may have triggered symptoms

In the event of a faint, carers need to know what to do:

- Lay the patient down flat
- Carry out simple first aid checks for breathing and circulation
- Think about safety, e.g. moving hot drinks
- Raise the patient's legs

Armed with this information, the need to call urgent medical attention can be avoided.

Constipation

According to estimates from the Sarah Matheson Trust, over 70% of MSA patients experience constipation. This is higher than in the palliative care patient group, of whom 50–60% will experience constipation, because of factors such as impaired nutrition and medication. The autonomic nerves promote peristalsis throughout the digestive tract (from lower end of the oesophagus, intestines and rectum).

Strategies to prevent constipation include:

- Dietary advice to maintain sufficient levels of fluids and fibre. This may require dietetic referral
- Daily use of stimulants and bulkers such as senna and fibogel to promote diminished peristalsis
- For some patients the most successful management may be a planned regime of suppositories or enemas

Speech and swallowing

Quiet voice that fatigues easily

Communication assessment may initially provide simple advice about reducing noise levels while talking (switching the television off, for example). Equipment such as alphabet boards, amplifiers or Lightwriters can be introduced to use when the voice fatigues; this will encourage their use as speech becomes less available.

Slurred speech

This speech pattern can be difficult to understand even with controlled breathing, which can slow down the pace of speech. Patients can be mistaken for sounding drunk and a credit-card-sized note explaining otherwise is useful in public. The same message on an answerphone can alert unfamiliar callers to the speech problem.

Complete loss of sound/speech production

The progression of speech problems may make complete loss of speech inevitable for some patients and this progression may be identified by a speech and language therapist. If this is a possibility it will necessitate immediate team attention. A multidisciplinary team that decides who and when to tell the patient this information will be better equipped to support patients and carers with the emotional consequences (isolation, frustration, fear and anxiety).

Difficulty swallowing

This may present as coughing or choking when eating or drinking, although up to a third of patients may aspirate silently (Smith and Bryan 1992). Dysphagia and dysarthria can occur independently in MSA, and speech problems are not an indicator of impaired swallow. Conversely, swallowing problems can occur without any speech problems. Videofluoroscopy examinations of swallow in MSA should be considered for most patients.

Management may include advice about swallow technique (see Chapter 9). Nutritional intake assessment from a dietician may warrant the introduction of supplements or alternative forms of feeding. Supplements need to be used cautiously with patients who have autonomic symptoms as the high sugar content of many supplements can exacerbate postural hypotension.

A gastrostomy tube is a successful way of providing good nutrition and hydration and reducing the risk of aspiration for people with MSA. In addition to reducing the number of hours spent each day trying to maintain a normal intake, it assists symptom control. This needs to be introduced at an appropriate time and discussed in relation to the patient's own expectations about their future and the value of such interventions.

Drooling

Drooling is thought to result from the reduced frequency of unconscious swallows rather than overproduction of saliva. The position of the head and neck means that saliva dribbles forward in the mouth, and reduced lip control contributes to the problem.

Management with medication such as atropine can cause problems with side effects such as hallucinations. Alternative management strategies include the use of a swallow reminder brooch, which produces a small bleep to remind the wearer to swallow.

A hand-held suction pump may be a better alternative than wiping the mouth with tissues. Occasionally the saliva can become thick and tenacious. This may be indicative of dehydration, mouth breathing or a chest infection. Pineapple juice or ice cubes may prove useful, together with addressing any of the suspected causes.

Bladder

Urgency frequency, urine infections

Continence is achievable for most patients with MSA. Most patients have incomplete bladder emptying. Bladder assessment should include a post-micturition residual volume to determine the presence of incomplete bladder emptying.

Intermittent self-catheterization is useful, if the residual volume is over 100 ml, together with drugs to improve detrusor stability, e.g. tolterodine. Once self-catheterization becomes difficult because of impaired movement, an indwelling catheter should be considered. A suprapubic catheter is preferable because of the lower rates of infection. There may be instances where a partner feels able to perform intermittent catheterization, but as this may be only one of many tasks they will undertake as a carer, their stress level and support should be considered before training begins.

Nocturia
Usually this is a problem for patients with postural hypotension. During the day, while upright, patients do not perfuse their kidneys well and do not produce much urine. This situation is reversed once the patient lies down to sleep. Emptying the bladder using intermittent catheterization just before going to sleep can help. The use of antidiuretic tablets such as desmopressin at night, to reduce urine production and therefore bladder filling, can also help to reduce the need to empty the bladder at night.

Cognition

Cognition is not significantly affected in MSA. In fact, the presence of significant cognitive change may suggest an alternative diagnosis, such as Lewy body disease, or an additional disease, such as dementia, occurring in conjunction with MSA (Wenning et al 2000).

Increased emotional response
Patients may cry or laugh very easily in situations that would previously have left them unmoved. On questioning, patients are clear that this emotional lability is not connected to either low mood or hysteria; this response can, however, be successfully managed with antidepressant medication.

Depression
Depression is more likely to occur in patients with MSA when they have previously experienced depression, for example postnatal depression. It is usually responsive to antidepressant treatment such as selective serotonin re-uptake inhibitors (SSRIs) (Stefanova et al 2000).

Sweating

Excessive sweating (hyperhidrosis) sometimes occurs as a precursor to losing the ability to sweat at all (anhidrosis). A tympanic thermometer should be used to record core temperature. This gives a more accurate reading of core body temperature, especially during sepsis or extremes of environmental temperature.

Breathing

Snoring and apnoea
Noisy snoring is associated with vocal cord paralysis. Apnoea occurs partly as a response to this airway obstruction together with changes to the central respiratory drive, which is under autonomic control. Snoring and apnoea can cause oxygen desaturation, creating a hangover-type feeling in the morning or increased daytime sleepiness.

A sleep study assessment of respiration can be useful in determining whether continuous positive airway pressure (CPAP) ventilation would be useful.

Stridor
Patients with stridor can also desaturate and this may require management with a tracheostomy. This has implications for care, as someone who can perform suction will need to be available 24 hours a day.

Inspiratory sighs
Although common, inspiratory sighs are not problematic.

Pain

Neck and shoulder pain
This coat-hanger pain is a symptom of postural hypotension.

Muscle pain and cramps
Muscle pain and cramps are probably due to muscle weakness or spasticity. Positional advice from a physiotherapist can ease muscle tone. Muscle relaxants, such as baclofen or valium, can be effective but may cause drowsiness. This may not be a problem if muscle relaxants are used overnight. Resistant pain may respond to neuropathic pain agents, such as amitriptyline or gabapentin.

Sleep disorders

Vivid dreams and restless sleep
REM sleep behaviour disorder is common in MSA (Plazzi et al 1998). Patients move about, shout out or talk during REM sleep when they should have relaxed muscle tone. This is often accompanied by vivid dreams that are described as lifelike. An explanation of this may be the best treatment for the patient.

The role of nurses

The unique feature about nurses is that they have direct contact with all services needed by someone with MSA: community nurses, ward nurses, outpatient nurses, nurse specialists, hospice nurses, continence nurses and research nurses (for patients who intend to have a brain postmortem examination). Nurses can be the wheels that keep these services working together with the patient and each other.

Although nurses are not the only professional group with good communication skills in combination with the nursing ethos of partnership, nurses make great advocates for patients. Preparing patients for bad news and dealing with its effects are inherent from nurse training. Finding or inspiring coping skills and accepting sad realities are also essential parts of the nurse's role.

The pathology of MSA lies in the area above the neck, but it is the problems below the waist that give the greatest concern to patients. Nurses can, at times, play down their role in bladder and bowel management but being dry and comfortable has an enormous impact on the quality of daily life. These practical skills place nurses in pole position to be key workers for patients with MSA.

The future

There is no doubt that MSA is a terrible disease and current treatment is less than effective. Until the encouraging volume of study and research provides preventive or curative treatments, palliative care must be the objective. Whilst treatment may have shortcomings there is no reason for care to be deficient. Neither kindness or compassion is a substitute for knowledgeable and organized care, but they are fundamental to its delivery.

The Sarah Matheson Trust

The Trust has published a short guide to MSA, available from: The Sarah Matheson Trust, Pickering Unit, St Mary's Hospital, Praed Street, London W2 1NY (www.msaweb.co.uk).

References

Ansorge O, Lees A J and Daniel S E (2002) The neuropathology and neurochemistry of multiple system atrophy. In: C Mathias and R Bannister (eds.) Autonomic Failure: A Textbook of Clinical Disorders of the Autonomic Nervous System, 4th edition. Oxford: Oxford University Press pp. 321–328.

Ben-Shlomo Y, Wenning G K, Tison F and Quinn N P (1997) Survival of patients with pathologically proven multiple system atrophy: a meta-analysis. Neurology 48(2): 384–393.

Bleasdale-Barr K and Mathias C (1998) Neck and other pains in autonomic failure; their association with orthostatic hypotension. Journal of the Royal Society of Medicine 91: 355–359.

Boesch S M, Wenning G K, Ransmayr G and Poewe W (2002) Dystonia in multiple system atrophy. Journal of Neurology, Neurosurgery and Psychiatry 72: 300–303.

Bradbury S and Eggleston C (1925) Postural hypotension: a report of three cases. American Heart Journal 1: 73–86.

Consensus statement on the definition of orthostatic hypotension, pure autonomic failure and multiple system atrophy (1996) Clinical Autonomic Research 6: 125–126.

Dejerine JJ and Thomas A (1900) L'atrophie olivo-ponto-cérébelleuse. Nouvelle Iconographie de la Salpêtrière, Paris, 13: 330–370.

Gilman S, Low P A, Quinn N, Albanese A, Ben-Shlomo Y, Fowler C J, Kaufmann H, Klockgether T, Lang A E, Lantos P L, Litvan I, Mathias C J, Oliver E, Robertson D, Schatz I and Wenning G K (1998) Consensus statement on the diagnosis of multisystem atrophy. American Autonomic Society and American Academy of Neurology. Clinical Autonomic Research 8(6): 359–362.

Graham J G and Oppenheimer D R (1969) Orthostatic hypotension and nicotine sensitivity in a case of multiple system atrophy. Journal of Neurology, Neurosurgery and Psychiatry 32: 28–34.

Mathias C and Bannister R (2002) Clinical features and evaluation of the primary chronic autonomic failure syndromes. In: C Mathias and R Bannister (eds.) Autonomic Failure: A Textbook of Clinical Disorders of the Autonomic Nervous System, 4th edition. Oxford: Oxford University Press pp. 307–316.

Mathais C (1998) Treatment of postural hypotension. Journal of Neurology, Neurosurgery and Psychiatry 65(3): 285–289.

Motor Neurone Disease Association (2001)

Muller J, Wenning G K, Jellinger K, McKee A, Poewe W and Litvan I (2000) Progression of Hoehn and Yahr stages in parkinsonian disorders. A clinicopathologic study. Neurology 55(6): 888–891.

Muller J, Wenning G K, Verny M, McKee A, Chaudhuri K R, Jellinger K, Poewe W and Litvan I (2001) Progression of dysarthria and dysphagia in postmortem–confirmed parkinsonian disorders. Archives of Neurology 58(2): 259–264.

Papp M I, Kahn J E and Lantos P L (1989) Glial cytoplasmic inclusions in the CNS of patients with multiple system atrophy. Journal of Neurological Science 94: 79–100.

Plazzi G, Cortelli P, Montagna P et al (1998) REM sleep behaviour disorder differentiates pure autonomic failure from multiple system atrophy. Journal of Neurology, Neurosurgery and Psychiatry 64: 683–685.

Quinn N (1989) Multiple system atrophy – the nature of the beast. Journal of Neurology, Neurosurgery and Psychiatry 52(Special Suppl): 78–89.

Quinn N (1993) The motor disorder of multiple system atrophy. Journal of Neurology, Neurosurgery and Psychiatry 56: 1239–1242.

Schrag A, Kingsley D, Phatouros C, Mathias C J, Lees A J, Daniel S E and Quinn N P (1998) Clinical usefulness of magnetic resonance imaging in multiple system atrophy. Journal of Neurology, Neurosurgery and Psychiatry 65: 65–71.

Schrag A, Ben-Shlomo Y and Quinn N P (2000) Cross sectional prevalence survey of idiopathic Parkinson's disease and parkinsonism in London. British Medical Journal 321: 21–22.

Shy G M and Drager G A (1960) A neurological syndrome associated with orthostatic hypotension. A clinical-pathological study. Archives of Neurology, 2: 511–527.

Smith C H and Bryan K L (1992) Speech and swallowing dysfunction in multisystem atrophy. Clinical Rehabilitation 6: 291–298.

Stefanova N, Seppi K Scherfler C, Puschban Z and Wenning G K (2000) Depression in alpha-synucleinopathies: prevalence, pathophysiology and treatment. Journal of Neural Transmission 60(Suppl): 335–343.

Swan L and Dupont J (1999) Multiple system atrophy. Physical Therapy 79: 488–494.

The Neurological Alliance (2003) Neurological Numbers. The Neurological Alliance: London.

Tison F, Yekhel Chrysostome V et al. (2002) Parkinsonism in multiple system atrophy: natural history, severity (UPDRS-III), and disability assessment compared with Parkinson's disease. Movement Disorders 17(4): 701–709.

van der Eecken H, Adams RD and van Bogaert L (1960) Striopallidal-nigral degeneration. An hitherto undescribed lesion in paralysis agitans. Journal of Neuropathology and Experimental Neurology 19: 159–161.

Wenning G K, Ben-Shlomo Y, Magalhaes M, Daniel S E and Quinn N P (1994) Clinical features and natural history of multiple system atrophy. Brain 117: 835–845.

Wenning G K, Ben-Shlomo Y, Hughes A, Daniel S E, Lees A and Quinn N P (2000) What clinical features are most useful to distinguish definite multiple system atrophy from Parkinson's disease? Journal of Neurology, Neurosurgery and Psychiatry 68: 434–440.

Wenning G K and Braune S (2001) Multiple system atrophy: pathophysiology and management. CNS Drugs 15(11): 839–852.

Wenning G K, Schlerfler C, Granata R, Bösch S, Verny M, Chaudhuri K R, Jellinger K, Poewe W and Litvan I (1999) Time course of symptomatic orthostatic hypotension and urinary incontinence in patients with postmortem confirmed parkinsonian syndromes. Journal of Neurology, Neurosurgery and Psychiatry 67: 620–623.

CHAPTER FOURTEEN

The Parkinson's Disease Society

BARBARA CORMIE

The Parkinson's Disease Society of the United Kingdom (PDS) was established in 1969 by a carer, Mali Jenkins, who was amazed to find no support available when her sister was diagnosed. The Society now has over 28,000 members and more than 300 branches and support groups throughout the UK. It is the *only* national organization working exclusively to help people with Parkinson's disease (PD), their families and friends. The Society's mission is the conquest of PD, and the alleviation of the distress it causes, through effective research, education, welfare and communication.

PDS activities

Helpline

The PDS runs a confidential helpline service, which can be called Monday to Friday, 9.30am–5.30pm (except bank holidays). The helpline is staffed by a team of nurses who provide support and information to anyone affected by PD. The staff can also inform on the location and availability of Parkinson's Disease Nurse Specialists (PDNSs).

Information and resources

The PDS can offer information and advice on a wide range of issues relating to PD, including health and social care, equipment, respite, employment rights, benefits and finance, insurance and driving.

The PDS also has many resources available for people with PD, their families and carers, and people working with them. These include information sheets, leaflets, booklets, audio cassettes and videos, covering all aspects of PD. The PDS also produces a quarterly colour magazine about PD and ways of coping with the condition. A full list of resources is available on the PDS's website (www.parkinsons.org.uk).

Education

Education and professional development underpin the work of the PDS. The PDS offers a variety of educational courses and initiatives on national, regional and local levels across the whole of the UK to cater for the needs of professionals and lay people.

Respite and holidays

Respite care and residential and nursing home care can be very important for people with PD. The PDS is involved in developing high standards of practice in all these areas. It can give information to people with PD, their carers and families, and refer them to appropriate schemes in their area.

Research

The PDS funds over 40 research projects in the UK, spending more than £2 million a year, as well as supporting the PDS Tissue Bank.

The PDS funds both medical and welfare research. Medical research is dedicated to finding the cause, cure and prevention of PD, and developing improvements in available treatments. Welfare research aims to develop models of good practice, looking at the management of PD and improving services.

The PDS's Tissue Bank is an internationally acclaimed research unit, largely funded by the PDS. Using donated tissue from people with and without PD, researchers at the centre are looking at the processes in the brain related to parkinsonism. The centre also supplies tissue to other researchers in the UK and throughout the world.

Campaigns

As the only UK charity dedicated to supporting all people with PD, the PDS is involved in policy, campaigning and parliamentary issues across the fields of science, health and social care, and is determined to promote change that will improve the lives of all those affected by PD.

Public relations

The PDS is recognized as the national voice of people with PD, and campaigns on their behalf. Using the media, advertising and information materials, the PDS is determined to improve the understanding of PD by the general public.

Field staff

The PDS has staff working across the UK. Their role is to promote the PDS's aims in their area, working with branches, families affected by PD and statutory and voluntary organizations. A key aim is ensuring that people with PD and their families have access to the best quality care and services at a local level. The field staff also encourage the development of branches or support groups to meet local needs, support these branches in their activities and encourage links with other branches and the PDS as a whole. They are also involved in welfare, education, information and fundraising activities within their area.

Local branches

There are over 300 branches and support groups across the UK. They are run by volunteers, often people who have PD and their families and carers. Each branch is different in the help that it offers, but generally they provide opportunities for mutual support and social activities through monthly meetings and practical help at a local level. Some branches also have community support workers who can make home visits to branch members and other people living with PD to give them information and support. The branches are also involved in fundraising and public awareness.

Parkinson's Disease Nurse Specialists

PDNSs are nurses specially trained in the management of PD. They offer information, support and advice to people with PD, their carers and families, and act as a link between other professionals. Some are hospital based, and others work in the community. Unfortunately, there are not yet PDNSs throughout the UK, but their numbers continue to grow.

The PDS was instrumental in developing the role of the PDNS and continues to facilitate and encourage the development of these posts.

Black and minority ethnic communities

The Outreach Service, with offices in Birmingham and Leicester, aims to assist people from minority ethnic communities affected by PD. The service employs outreach workers. Their role is to provide information, advice and resources on PD and on the help available from other agencies, including Social Services, thus enabling clients and carers to make informed decisions about the care options available to them. They also work with other agencies to organize awareness and information days, to raise awareness within the black and minority ethnic communities. They can provide bilingual support in a number of Asian languages.

YAPP&Rs

YAPP&Rs (Young Alert Parkinson's, Partners and Relatives) is the PDS's special interest group for younger people with PD (i.e. of working age) and their families. YAPP&Rs members offer each other mutual support through their network of support groups, their magazine, the *YAPmag*, and phone calls. Every 2 years they organize a national conference held over a weekend.

SPRING

The Special Parkinson's Research Interest Group (SPRING) is a special interest group within the PDS whose focus is medical research. Members of SPRING help the PDS to increase the profile of medical research and raise funds to support projects throughout the UK.

Fundraising

The PDS could not function without money. The Fundraising Department works extremely hard to raise money to fund all the PDS's services. In an increasingly difficult environment, the PDS appreciates the generous support it receives from all its members and supporters.

Contact details

Parkinson's Disease Society (Registered Charity No. 258197)
215 Vauxhall Bridge Road, London, SW1V 1EJ.
Tel 020 7931 8080, Fax 020 7233 9908

E-mail enquiries@parkinsons.org.uk

Website www.parkinsons.org.uk (includes details of all PDS resources)

Helpline (available Monday–Friday (except Bank Holidays), 9.30am–5.30pm). Freephone 0808 800 0303.
Textphone (Minicom) 020 7963 9380

CHAPTER FIFTEEN

The Parkinson's Disease Nurse Specialist Association

KAREN VERNON

Background

The first Parkinson's disease Nurse Specialist (PDNS) was appointed in Cornwall in 1989. During the early 1990s, the number of PDNSs remained few and the posts often existed in isolation, with little or no opportunity for the nurses to interact with one another. It was against this background that the Royal College of Nursing facilitated the development of a working party of PDNSs. The group was elected from practising PDNSs and was endorsed by the then Chief Nurse for England, Dame Yvonne Moores. Following the success of this group it was decided that an independent, national representative group of PDNSs be formed and in 1999 the Parkinson's Disease Nurse Specialist Association (PDNSA) was established.

Aims of the PDNSA

From its outset, the main aim of the PDNSA has been to act as a national resource and network for PDNSs and for other health and social care professionals who deal with people with Parkinson's disease (PD). The association encourages sharing of knowledge, expertise and examples of best practice about PD and its management. It is also increasingly becoming a point of reference for the Department of Health and other statutory bodies for a wide variety of issues that influence the profession of nursing as a whole, and specifically PD nursing.

The PDNSA committee

The current executive committee of the PDNSA consists of eight elected

PDNSs who provide a representative body of nurses working within the field of PD. The current offices within the committee are:

- Chair
- Vice chair
- Secretary
- Treasurer
- Membership officer
- Educational officer
- Website officer
- International representative
- Research officer

A member of the committee is also the editor of the PDNSA's quarterly newsletter, the *Transmitter*, and another committee member oversees the organization of the PDNSA's annual conference.

When a committee vacancy occurs, nurses who have been members of the PDNSA for at least 1 year can put themselves forward for election. Dependent upon the number of applicants for the vacancy, the membership then vote for who they feel would best represent their interests. Committee members then serve a 2-year term of office, after which they can stand for re-election.

PDNSA membership

Membership of the PDNSA is open to all PDNSs and other professionals from health and social care who deal with or have an interest in the management and associated issues of PD.

There are two types of membership available: full or associate. Membership type is dependent upon the person's role and their amount of contact with people with PD. There is a small membership fee, for which the members currently receive:

- A quarterly newsletter – *Transmitter*
- Educational resources
- Reduced fees for the annual PDNSA conference
- Access to the members-only section on the PDNSA website (see below)
- Access to PDNSA bursary for education, research or service development

As the membership expands and the association develops, it is envisaged that membership benefits will continue to increase. Overseas membership is available to those working within the field of PD, with many of the same benefits being available. The advent of the PDNSA website will allow overseas members to become active voices of the membership.

PDNSA publications

The PDNSA has been involved with the production of a document which has looked at the role of the PDNSs. The latest edition of the document entitled *The Role of the Parkinson's Disease Nurse Specialist* was published in 2001. The aim of this document is to highlight the increasing importance of this specialist role and it builds upon the inaugural document by incorporating recent changes within the clinical grading for nurse specialists and the ever-expanding role of the PDNS. The document also provides a blueprint for recommendations, qualifications and skills for the role and the responsibilities of the PDNS. The PDNSA is currently involved in developing similar documents for Scotland, Wales and Northern Ireland, which will address specific issues for PDNSs within these countries.

There is a recently completed publication about surgery for PD patients (Stross et al 2004). The PDNSA worked with, and supported, a steering group of nurses working within this aspect of PD nursing. Ongoing joint ventures with PDNSA members either on an individual basis or with a group of members will hopefully lead to further publications.

Transmitter

This is a quarterly newsletter produced and edited by the PDNSA committee and it is an important aspect of the association's work, as it is an effective means of ensuring dissemination of information to all members. Its contents include:

- Articles written by the association's members
- Articles by guest writers
- Reflection upon conferences and study days
- PDNSA current activities

The newsletter tries to reflect the current national and international influences on PD nursing.

Website

The PDNSA has developed a website (www.pdnsa.org.uk). The website contains the following material:

- A section for PDNSA members that is password protected. This section contains educational material such as information on deep brain stimulation and allows members to interact online. This section of the website has only recently been developed but it is hoped that it will become an important resource for all PDNSs
- Back copies of *Transmitter*
- Links to other associated websites such as the Parkinson's Disease Society
- A section for joining the PDNSA
- A section for registering for the annual PDNSA conference
- Abstracts from previous conferences

Development of the website is ongoing.

Annual conference

The PDNSA holds an annual 2-day conference which is open to members and non-members. Whilst the themes and topics change on a yearly basis, the conference tries to concentrate on a particular aspect of PD for the first day, and looks at professional and governmental issues affecting healthcare on the second. These talks take place in both platform presentations and workshop format to allow for interaction from the delegates. Topics that have been presented at conference include deep brain stimulation, palliative care and spirituality in PD, dementia and PD, National Service Frameworks and how they affect PD healthcare, clinical governance and nurse prescribing, to name a few. Information about the forthcoming PDNSA conference is available on the PDNSA website.

Education

Education has been identified as an important aspect of the role of the PDNSA both from a professional and personal perspective of PDNSs. In a survey of PDNSA members in 2002, education of self and of others featured very prominently in the survey results. The identification of an educational officer has allowed the PDNSA to concentrate upon the specific educational needs of the PDNSs and identify and develop ways in which to support them.

One way has been for the PDNSA to develop educational resources, available to full members of the association, which can act as a point of reference or guidance to PDNSs, particularly those new to the role. Current ideas for educational resources include information about:

- Audit tools
- Membership guidelines
- Lone worker policy
- Assessment tools
- Guidance for nurses using apomorphine
- Supplementary nurse prescribing
- Clinical management plans

Nurse prescribing will potentially have a great impact upon the roles of PDNSs and consequently information on supplementary prescribing is to be a major educational resource. A section on drug protocols for implementation at a local level has recently been included.

The development of educational resources is an ongoing project of the PDNSA and reflects the changing demands on nurse specialist roles from both a professional and a governmental perspective.

Professional development and retention is a concern amongst specialist practitioners and the PDNSA recognizes that an important aspect of its role is to provide support to its members in a variety of ways. In the survey undertaken for the PDNSA of its members in 2002, important influences on the developing roles of the PDNS were elicited. The concerns expressed by the members have acted as an action plan for the association in how to channel future activities and, in doing so, how to address some of these concerns and provide support to all PDNSs.

Research

The PDNSA has recently appointed a research officer to the committee and established a research bursary. The bursary is available to all PDNSA members and applicants should submit their proposals to the committee for consideration. It is hoped that the bursary will encourage more nurses to undertake nursing research.

Conclusion

The role of the PDNS is diverse and the practitioners who fulfil this role are specialist professionals who exercise high levels of judgement, discretion and decision-making in clinical care. They are able to monitor and improve standards of care through supervision of practice and clinical audit. They provide skilled professional leadership and develop nursing practice through research, teaching and supporting colleagues from other disciplines.

Often owing to constraints of time, the members of the PDNSA are limited in their ability to meet and influence activity for PDNSs as a collective force. Forming links with national and international statutory bodies, as well as health and social care personnel and the voluntary sector, is seen as essential in continuing to raise the profile of PDNSs. The PDNSA provides the professional voice for these practitioners and, in turn, continues to ensure that these highly skilled professionals are supported and listened to.

CHAPTER SIXTEEN

Future developments in the treatment of Parkinson's disease

PETER HAGELL

The initial response to symptomatic dopaminergic drug therapy for Parkinson's disease (PD) is often excellent. However, after some years of treatment most patients develop complications of therapy, such as motor, autonomic and psychiatric problems. The main motor complications are diurnal fluctuations and dyskinesias (Quinn 1998). With time, treatment complications increase in severity and make it difficult to provide an optimal drug therapy (Lang and Lozano 1998; Quinn 1998). The need for novel therapeutic interventions that are able to offer relief from the underlying disease as well as from long-term complications is thus apparent. In this respect, alternative promising dopaminergic (DA-ergic) and non-DA-ergic compounds, as well as neurosurgical interventions, have recently caused great interest (Olanow et al 2001). The currently available therapeutic options are symptomatic, by compensating either for the deficit in striatal dopamine (DA) transmission or for the secondary imbalance downstream in the basal ganglia, but recent advances include new and fundamentally different approaches to the treatment of PD that go beyond the current therapeutic paradigm. This chapter focuses on two such possibilities: first, to repair the affected brain by replacing lost neurons with new ones and, second, to slow or halt the underlying disease process.

Cell replacement

The basic principle of cell replacement therapy in PD is to replace lost DA neurons with new ones, thereby restoring striatal DA-ergic transmission. The idea of transplanting neural tissue is not new, and the first attempts took place more than a century ago. Almost nine decades later, the observation that grafted embryonic DA-ergic tissue can survive and reverse experimentally induced parkinsonism in the rat implied that if the brain can be repaired and neurological deficits can be reversed in experimental animals, it should also be possible to achieve this in human disease

(Dunnett and Björklund 1994). Since then, there have been clinical trials using various sources of graft tissue (allogeneic, autogeneic and xenogeneic tissue). However, only use of allografts of human ventral mesencephalon (VM) tissue harvested from embryos following elective abortions has yielded consistent graft survival and clinical benefits (Lindvall 1994; Barker 2002; Lindvall and Hagell 2002).

The first clinical transplantation trials with intrastriatal grafts of allogeneic DA-rich tissue from embryonic VM were performed in the late 1980s. The first evidence for survival of DA-ergic neurons in the grafts, associated with substantial clinical improvement, were provided in 1990 by demonstration of an increased postoperative striatal uptake of 6-L-[^{18}F]-fluorodopa (FD), a measure of DA terminal function, using positron emission tomography (PET) (Lindvall et al 1990). Subsequent histopathological studies in patients with positive postoperative FD PET findings who died about 18 months after transplantation showed between 80,000 and 135,000 surviving DA-ergic neurons in each putamen (Kordower et al 1995, 1998). Neuritic outgrowth from the grafted neurons with synaptic graft-to-host connections and re-innervation of the target area was found. Subsequent studies have shown that DA-rich grafts are able also to restore spontaneous and drug-induced synaptic DA release (Piccini et al 1999), and integrate functionally with the host basal ganglia–thalamo–cortical circuit, which seems necessary for substantial clinical improvement (Piccini et al 2000).

Several independent open-label clinical trials have shown that intrastriatal DA-ergic grafts of primary human embryonic VM tissue can survive and induce symptomatic relief (Lindvall and Hagell 2000, 2002). These trials have typically shown a restoration from about 30% of the normal putamen FD PET uptake preoperatively to about 50% during the second postoperative year. Most of the patients with surviving grafts have gradually, over 6–24 months, experienced a greater amount of time spent in the 'on' phase, improved PD symptoms in the 'off' phase, and reduced drug requirement. By the second postoperative year, overall symptomatic relief, as assessed by the Unified Parkinson's Disease Rating Scale (UPDRS) motor score, has typically been between 30 and 40%. In the best cases, 'off' phases have disappeared and patients have been able to stop medication and resume full-time work. Sustained graft viability, clinical benefit, and graft-derived DA release have been reported for up to 10 years after transplantation (Piccini et al 1999). However, there is substantial variation in the magnitude of symptomatic relief among patients and, even in the best cases, recovery has been incomplete.

In 2001, the first double-blind, placebo-controlled trial showed a generally more modest, but statistically significant, symptomatic response (Freed et al 2001). The procedure employed in this trial differed from most open-label trials in several central respects, including amount and preparation of graft tissue, immunosuppression and surgical technique (Dunnett et al 2001). Nevertheless, this study provides the first direct evidence of a specific graft-induced improvement, distinguishable from that of sham surgery. More recently, a second double-blind, placebo-controlled trial failed to demonstrate statistically significant differences between grafted patients and those undergoing sham surgery (Olanow et al 2003). A significant treatment effect was, however, seen in grafted patients with less severe preoperative disease.

The effect on dyskinesias following transplantation has been inconsistent in open-label trials, with reported increases as well as decreases (Lindvall and Hagell 2000). In the double-blind trial by Freed et al (2001), 15% of the grafted patients developed severe postoperative dyskinesias in the 'off' phase. 'Off' phase dyskinesias have also been described by other groups, albeit generally mild (Cenci and Hagell in press). The mechanism behind this side effect is obscure. Postoperative 'off' phase dyskinesias have thus typically not been related to the magnitude of graft-derived DA-ergic re-innervation or symptomatic relief (Hagell et al 2002a; Olanow et al 2003). However, PET findings have indicated that an unbalanced putaminal DA-ergic function may contribute (Ma et al 2002). Other factors that may contribute include graft composition, placement and integration, as well as host immune reactions (Cenci and Hagell in press).

Although clinical trials performed thus far have provided proof of concept for the cell replacement strategy in PD, it seems unlikely that transplantation of primary human embryonic VM tissue can become a feasible clinical therapy. In addition to ethical concerns relating to the use of human tissue from aborted embryos, several obstacles exist. First, a major problem is the need for multiple donors for each patient (Hagell and Brundin 2001; Björklund et al 2003), which makes it difficult to obtain sufficient donor tissue on a regular basis. Second, recent observations (Hagell et al 2002a) indicate a need for better standardization of graft tissue (Isacson et al 2003). Third, the symptomatic efficacy and the variability in outcome need to be improved (Björklund et al 2003). Finally, the reason(s) for the development of postoperative dyskinesias in some patients must be elucidated so that this side effect can be avoided (Cenci and Hagell in press). Until these problems have been resolved, cell replacement therapy will not be suitable for large-scale clinical application. Stem cells may offer solutions to current challenges (Freed 2002; Björklund et al 2003; Isacson et al 2003).

Stem cells

During recent years the stem cell technique has been of enormous interest in the neuroscience community, as well as in the public media, because of the potential therapeutic implications for incurable disorders, such as PD (Lindvall and Hagell 2002; Steindler and Pincus 2002; Barker et al 2003). Stem cells are characterized by multipotency (the ability to develop into different types of cells) and self-renewal (activation results in the designated cell type, plus a new stem cell) (Armstrong and Svendsen 2000).

Efforts to understand, control and use stem cells for therapeutic purposes are intense and knowledge is increasing rapidly. Different potential sources of stem cells for transplantation in PD have emerged, e.g. DA-ergic precursors from the embryonic brain, embryonic stem cells and stem cells harvested from adult tissues, such as bone marrow or brain. Various approaches can be envisaged regarding the use of such cells for brain restoration in PD. The first is that stem cells are predifferentiated to DA neurons in the laboratory and then implanted into the denervated striatum in a manner similar to that used in current clinical transplantation trials (Studer et al 1998; Kim et al 2002). The important differences, however, are that stem cells could become an unlimited source of DA neurons, and that the number and composition of implanted cells would be known and controllable. Alternatively, stem cells could be implanted directly and then undergo differentiation in the brain (Björklund et al 2002). Hypothetically, this could result in better integration and perhaps allow reconstruction of the nigrostriatal system. Third, the finding that the adult human brain hosts neural stem cells (Kukekov et al 1999) has raised the possibility that the patient's own neural stem cells could be taken out, predifferentiated in vitro, and reimplanted. Fourth, while challenged (Ying et al 2002), another intriguing possibility is suggested by observations indicating that bone marrow stem cells may migrate to the CNS and differentiate into neuronal cells (Mezey et al 2000). If confirmed, this could mean that it would be possible to repair brain lesions by use of bone marrow stem cells or by manipulation of bone marrow to induce stem cell migration and differentiation. Finally, brain self-repair could hypothetically also be promoted by administration of selective neuropoietins, i.e. compounds triggering repair processes by intrinsic stem cells (Steindler and Pincus 2002).

However, several fundamental issues need to be resolved before any of these options can be considered for clinical trials (Barker 2002; Freed 2002; Lindvall and Hagell 2002; Steindler and Pincus 2002). First, studies performed so far have mainly been conducted in rodents and little is known about how well these data translate into humans. Second, safety issues related to potential tumour formation need to be eliminated. Third, DA neurons derived from stem cells have, in general, thus far shown relatively poor survival after transplantation and little has been documented regarding long-term survival. It is also unclear if these cells display the necessary functional characteristics after grafting. This should be put in the context of requirements that, based on results from clinical trials and animal models using primary embryonic donor tissue, have to be fulfilled in order for grafts to induce clinically valuable improvements. These include sufficient graft survival, functional and structural integration with host brain circuitries, effective intrastriatal graft-derived DA release and capacity to induce functional recovery in animal PD models. With few exceptions (Björklund et al 2002; Kim et al 2002), these requirements are yet to be met by the stem cell technique.

Neuroprotection

An attractive approach to the treatment of PD is to slow or, ultimately, halt the disease process. Because the neurodegenerative process in PD probably involves a series of interrelated events, such as oxidative stress, mitochondrial dysfunction and excitotoxicity, neuroprotection may be possible through intervening with any of these events (Dunnett and Björklund 1999). Furthermore, since DA neurodegeneration appears to be a slow process, with neurons being progressively dysfunctional for some time before actually dying, there should also be room for delaying cell death and restoring neuronal function (Dunnett and Björklund 1999). This section reviews some of the available and emerging potential neuroprotective strategies.

Potential neuroprotective effects of currently available treatments

The observation that selegiline-mediated inhibition of monoaminoxidase B (MAOB) prevents 1-methyl-4-phenyl-1,2,3,6-tetrahydropyridine (MPTP)-induced nigral cell death in animal models raised the possibility that selegiline may be able to provide neuroprotection in PD. Initial clinical trials appeared encouraging, with selegiline-treated patients displaying slower clinical progression than those not treated with selegiline (Parkinson Study Group 1989; Tetrud and Langston 1989). However, these observations have subsequently proved inconclusive because of the symptomatic effects of selegiline, and its possible neuroprotective features remain controversial (Koller 1998; Shoulson et al 1998; Olanow et al 2001). Nonetheless, selegiline can be neuroprotective in laboratory models, although this effect is probably not due to MAOB inhibition or selegiline per se but to inhibition of apoptotic (programmed) cell death and the selegiline metabolite desmethylselegiline (Tatton and Greenwood 1991; Mytilineou et al 1997; Olanow et al 2001).

More recently, interest has turned toward DA agonists as possible neuroprotective agents by exertion of, for example, presynaptic DA autoreceptor stimulation with reduced DA turnover, and antioxidative free-radical scavenging effects (Olanow et al 1998). Evidence for putative neuroprotective actions of DA agonists has been obtained in several laboratory models (Olanow et al 1998). Apomorphine, for example, can act as a potent free-radical scavenger (Gassen et al 1996), and provide significant protection against MPTP-induced nigrostriatal DA-ergic cell loss in mice (Grünblatt et al 1999). Recent data suggest that these neuroprotective effects may be mediated by an apomorphine-induced astrocyte expression of neurotrophic factors (Ohta et al 2000). It remains to be determined whether apomorphine is neuroprotective in PD patients treated with clinically applied doses (Hagell and Odin 2001). However, recent clinical trials have implied possible neuroprotective effects of newer DA agonists. For example, in a 46-month prospective follow-up of 82 patients with early PD treated with either levodopa or the DA agonist pramipexole, striatal uptake of the DA transporter ligand β-CIT, as measured using SPECT, was found to decrease more rapidly in patients started on levodopa (25.5% decrease), compared with those initiating treatment with pramipexole (16% decrease) (Parkinson Study Group 2002). Similar findings, using FD PET, have also been presented in favour of initial treatment with ropinirole compared to levodopa (Whone et al 2003). However, interpretation of these observations remains ambiguous (Morrish 2002, 2003; Ahlskog 2003). For example, while differences in the neuroimaging outcomes were found between study drugs in both trials, these were not mirrored in terms of patients' clinical progression. Furthermore, the possibility that the observed differences are due to a pharmacological interaction between study drugs and imaging ligands cannot be ruled out. Thus current data do not provide unequivocal evidence for clinical neuroprotective effects of DA-agonists.

One consequence of the imbalance in the basal ganglia circuitry in PD is an overactivation of glutamatergic projections from the subthalamic nucleus (STN) to, for example, globus pallidus and the substantia nigra (SN), which may contribute to neurodegeneration through excitotoxicity. It has thus been speculated that glutamate-inhibiting drugs and deep brain stimulation (DBS) of the STN may exert neuroprotective effects (Rodriguez et al 1998). Although it is yet to be demonstrated in humans, data from neurosurgical deactivation of the STN in a rat PD model have suggested such an effect (Piallat et al 1999). Furthermore, administration of the glutamate release-inhibitor riluzole to monkeys with MPTP-induced parkinsonism has shown symptomatic as well as neuroprotective effects (Obinu et al 2002). However, initial clinical trials have failed to demonstrate any advantages, or signs of neuroprotective effects, with riluzole over placebo in early PD (Rascol et al 2002).

Emerging neuroprotective strategies

Neurotrophic factors are proteins that are important for neuronal development and regeneration after injury. In PD, glial cell line derived neurotrophic factor (GDNF) has shown the most promising results. Animal studies in various species have shown that GDNF can not only exert neuroprotective effects on nigrostriatal DA neurons, but also stimulate axonal growth and DA turnover and function in residual neurons (Björklund et al 1997; Lapchak and Araujo 2001). This prompted the initiation of a double-blind clinical trial with monthly intraventricular injections of GDNF or placebo (Nutt et al 2003). No clinical improvements were observed, but adverse events such as nausea, vomiting, anorexia and paresthesias (in particular L'hermitte's sign) were common in GDNF-treated patients. Autopsy data from one patient who died for unrelated reasons (Kordower et al 1999) showed that only negligible levels of GDNF reached nigral neurons and failed to induce DA-ergic regeneration. The lack of neurotrophic or clinical effects was probably due to the fact that neurotrophic molecules are capable of tissue penetration only to a limited extent (Emborg et al 2001), and side effects may have resulted from the wide dispersal of GDNF throughout the CNS. Thus, in order for this modality of treatment to succeed, local intraparenchymal administration within or close to the target area(s) appears necessary. Intraputaminal infusion of GDNF was recently studied in five patients with advanced PD (Gill et al 2003). At 1 year, parkinsonian symptoms were improved by 39% and putaminal FD PET showed a 28% increase in the region around the infusion catheter after 18 months. Smaller increases in FD PET uptake were also observed in the SN. Adverse events were relatively few and described as mild. The mechanisms behind the observed effects are yet to be established, but may involve a combined protective and regenerative or DA-release stimulating effect. These observations support the notion that GDNF may be safely used in PD if supplied locally in the brain area of interest.

Gene therapy, by which lengths of DNA are placed into a carrying vector that is introduced into cells, provides a means of delivering, for example, neurotrophic factors, in a site-specific fashion using one of two strategies (Tenenbaum et al 2002). In ex vivo gene therapy, cells are genetically modified in culture to express the desired molecule and are then grafted to the site of interest in the recipient brain. Using in vivo gene therapy, the host cells themselves are genetically modified by vectors that are stereotaxically introduced into the desired target area(s) where they deliver genes that encode for the therapeutic molecule.

Using in vivo lentivirus gene therapy, Kordower et al (2000) delivered GDNF into the striatum and SN of aged monkeys with nigrostriatal degeneration similar to that in early PD, and of young adult animals with prominent hemiparkinsonism following unilateral MPTP injections. GDNF reversed nigrostriatal degeneration in aged monkeys and improved parkinsonism in MPTP-lesioned young monkeys. Autopsy revealed sparing of nigral DA neurons and partial preservation of striatal DA innervation in GDNF-treated monkeys. While these observations are promising and point to the possibility of a future neuroprotective therapy in PD, several issues remain to be resolved before the initiation of clinical trials, including safety issues related to viral transfection and development of systems that make it possible to titrate and shut off the GDNF gene expression (Björklund and Lindvall 2000). One ex vivo gene therapeutic approach that could be advantageous from a safety perspective is implantation of genetically engineered cells (for production of GDNF, for example) encapsulated in a membrane that allows inward diffusion of nutrients and outward diffusion of therapeutic molecules (Bensadoun et al 2001). In case of adverse events, such encapsulated cells could be removed surgically. Initial clinical trials using this technique in amyotrophic lateral sclerosis have been performed (Aebischer et al 1996), and animal experiments in PD models have shown promising results, with clinical trials under consideration (Bensadoun et al. 2001).

Prospects and implications

Current scientific developments are impressive, rapid and promising, and indicate that it may soon be possible to offer therapeutic strategies that go well beyond those available today. However, much work remains before approaches such as stem cell based therapy and in vivo gene transfer can be considered clinically feasible. In the meantime, issues going beyond biological complexity will also need to be considered.

There is currently an increasing emphasis on evidence-based medicine. One fundamental question is by what means and to what degree of objectivity and accuracy we are able to measure outcomes of clinical trials. In this respect, emerging therapeutic principles such as neuroprotective and restorative interventions may be more challenging than current symptomatic drug therapies. In order to assess the effects of such approaches we will thus need assessment tools that cover a broad spectrum of consequences of the disease with sufficient accuracy. Such tools should be feasible and not introduce unnecessary burdens for patient and investigator. In order to fulfil these needs, the methods used should be relevant, well defined, reliable, valid and responsive (Hobart et al 1996; Wright 1997). Very few currently available outcome measures in PD meet such criteria (Hagell 2002; Holloway and Dick 2002). The increasing demands for patient-reported outcomes have, for example, yet to be coupled with the development of high quality measures in PD. For instance, while the

PD-specific health status questionnaire PDQ-39 has gained widespread use, its measurement validity still appears ambiguous and recent data indicate that it is not suitable for patients in early stages of the disease (Hagell et al 2003), a major target group for neuroprotective trials (Olanow et al 2001).

Given the current escalating healthcare expenditures, shrinking resources and rising life expectancy, health economic aspects of disease and therapy are likely to become increasingly important as new and potentially costly treatments, such as those discussed here, are developed. As an illustration, Siderowf and co-workers (1998) in the US found indications of higher costs, but also better effectiveness, of pramipexole compared to baseline PD management, whereas pallidotomy would reach the same cost-effectiveness only if procedure costs were reduced by two-thirds or if the postoperative utility was equivalent to being restored to normal health. In order to evaluate the economic implications of new interventions, it is important to consider the current economic impact of the disease. Health economic studies on the cost of PD have begun to emerge (Scheife et al 2000; Hagell et al 2002b) and provide valuable baseline data for future health economic evaluations of novel therapeutic interventions. These studies indicate that PD causes a considerable societal burden although direct medical costs often do not dominate, thus implying that there should be considerable room for novel approaches to prove cost-effective given sufficient ability to offer long-term relief and independence.

Conclusions

Current information technologies allow for rapid dissemination of scientific advances, often in an enthusiastic and oversimplified manner, leaving patients and families with unrealistic hopes for immediate help. Therefore, it is of paramount importance for nurses and other clinicians to be able to provide accurate and balanced information regarding scientific advances and clinical prospects. It must, for example, be emphasized that our current understanding of emerging interventions for PD is in great need of improvement and clinical applications are, in most instances, remote. Progress toward the clinic should be made with great care and, once appropriate, therapeutic trials should be conducted according to highest standards.

Key points

- Fundamentally novel approaches to the treatment of PD, such as restoration of dopamine transmission and slowing of the underlying disease process, are emerging

- Clinical neural transplantation trials using primary human embryonic tissue have been promising but the need for multiple donors, variable clinical outcome and unexpected side effects makes further developments necessary before cell transplantation can become clinically feasible
- The stem cell technique may provide the means necessary for a future dopamine cell replacement therapy for PD, but several fundamental biological issues remain to be resolved before clinical trials can commence
- Neuroprotective effects of currently available treatments, for example selegiline, dopamine agonists and deep brain stimulation, need to be firmly demonstrated
- Neurotrophic factors, such as GDNF, may provide effective neuroprotection in PD but clinical applications are in their infancy
- In parallel with biotechnological advancements, efforts should be made to improve methods of outcomes measurement in order to answer currently unmet needs and allow firm interpretation of trial results

Acknowledgements

The author's own work in this field has been supported by the Swedish Medical Research Council, the Kock Foundation, the Wiberg Foundation, the King Gustav V and Queen Victoria Foundation, the Skane County Council Research and Development Foundation and the Söderberg Foundation. The author wishes to thank O Lindvall, H Widner and P Brundin for valuable discussions.

References

Aebischer P, Schluep M, Deglon N, Joseph J M, Hirt L, Heyd B, Goddard M, Hammang J P, Zurn A D, Kato A C, Regli F and Baetge E E (1996) Intrathecal delivery of CNTF using encapsulated genetically modified xenogeneic cells in amyotrophic lateral sclerosis patients. Nature Medicine 2: 696–699.

Ahlskog J E (2003) Slowing Parkinson's disease progression: recent dopamine agonist trials. Neurology 60: 381–389.

Armstrong R J E and Svendsen C N (2000) Neural stem cells: from cell biology to cell replacement. Cell Transplantation 9: 139–152.

Barker R A (2002) Repairing the brain in Parkinson's disease: Where next? Movement Disorders 17: 233–241.

Barker R A, Jain M, Armstrong R J E and Caldwell M A (2003) Stem cells and neurological disease. Journal of Neurology, Neurosurgery and Psychiatry 74: 553–557.

Bensadoun J C, Widmer H R, Zurn A D and Aebischer P (2001) Polymer-encapsulated cells as a tool for drug delivery and neural transplantation in Parkinson's disease. In: J K Krauss and J Jankovic (eds.) Surgery for Parkinson's Disease and Movement Disorders. Philadelphia: Lippincott Williams and Wilkins pp. 245–251.

Björklund A and Lindvall O (2000) Parkinson disease gene therapy moves toward the clinic. Nature Medicine 6: 1207–1208.

Björklund A, Rosenbald C, Winkler C and Kirik D (1997) Studies on neuroprotective and regenerative effects of GDNF in a partial lesion model of Parkinson's disease. Neurobiology of Disease 4: 186–200.

Bjorklund A, Dunnett S B, Brundin P, Stoessl A J, Freed C R, Breeze R E, Levivier M, Peschanski M, Studer L and Barker R (2003) Neural transplantation for the treatment of Parkinson's disease. Lancet Neurology 2: 437–445.

Björklund L M, Sanchez-Pernaute R, Chung S, Andersson T, Chen I Y, McNaught K S, Brownell A L, Jenkins B G, Wahlestedt C, Kim K S and Isacson O (2002) Embryonic stem cells develop into functional dopaminergic neurons after transplantation in a Parkinson rat model. Proceedings of the National Academy of Sciences of the United States of America 99: 2344–2349.

Cenci M A and Hagell P (in press) Dyskinesias and neural grafting in Parkinson's disease. In: W C Olanow and P Brundin (eds.) Restorative Therapies in Parkinson's Disease. New York: Kluwer Academic/Plenum Publishers.

Dunnett S B and Björklund A (1994) Introduction. In: S B Dunnett, A Björklund (eds.) Functional Neural Transplantation. New York: Raven Press Ltd pp. 1–7.

Dunnett S B and Björklund A (1999) Prospects for new restorative and neuroprotective treatments in Parkinson's disease. Nature 399(suppl): A32–39.

Dunnett S B, Björklund A and Lindvall O (2001) Cell therapy in Parkinson's disease – stop or go? Nature Reviews. Neuroscience 2: 365–369.

Emborg M E, Deglon N, Leventhal L, Aebischer P and Kordower J H (2001) Viral vector-mediated gene therapy for Parkinson's disease. Clinical Neuroscience Research 1: 496–506.

Freed C R (2002) Will embryonic stem cells be a useful source of dopamine neurons for transplant into patients with Parkinson's disease? Proceedings of the National Academy of Sciences of the United States of America 99: 1755–1757.

Freed C R, Greene P E, Breeze R E, Tsai W Y, DuMouchel W, Kao R, Dillon S, Winfield H, Culver S, Trojanowski J Q, Eidelberg D and Fahn S (2001) Transplantation of embryonic dopamine neurons for severe Parkinson's disease. New England Journal of Medicine 344: 710–719.

Gassen M, Glinka Y, Pinchasi B and Youdim M B (1996) Apomorphine is a highly potent free radical scavenger in rat brain mitochondrial fraction. European Journal of Pharmacology 308: 219–226.

Gill S S, Patel N K, Hotton G R, O'Sullivan K, McCarter R, Bunnage M, Brooks D J, Svendsen C N and Heywood P (2003) Direct brain infusion of glial cell line-derived neurotrophic factor in Parkinson's disease. Nature Medicine 9: 589–595.

Grünblatt E, Mandel S, Berkuzki T and Youdim M B (1999) Apomorphine protects against MPTP-induced neurotoxicity in mice. Movement Disorders 14: 612–618.

Hagell P and Brundin P (2001) Cell survival and clinical outcome following intrastriatal transplantation in Parkinson's disease. Journal of Neuropathology and Experimental Neurology 60: 741–752.

Hagell P and Odin P (2001) Apomorphine in the treatment of Parkinson's disease. Journal of Neuroscience Nursing 33: 21–38.

Hagell P, Piccini P, Björklund A, Brundin P, Rehncrona S, Widner H, Crabb L, Pavese N, Oertel W H, Quinn N, Brooks D J and Lindvall O (2002a) Dyskinesias following neural transplantation in Parkinson's disease. Nature Neuroscience 5: 627–628.

Hagell P, Nordling S, Reimer J, Grabowski M and Persson U (2002b) Resource use and costs in a Swedish cohort of patients with Parkinson's disease. Movement Disorders 17: 1213–1220.

Hagell P, Whalley D, McKenna S P and Lindvall O (2003) Health status measurement in Parkinson's disease: validity of the PDQ-39 and Nottingham Health Profile. Movement Disorders 18: 773–783.

Hagell P (2002) Assessment of graft effects and function in cell replacement therapy for Parkinson's disease [dissertation]. Lund, Sweden: Lund University, 2002.

Hobart J C, Lamping D L and Thompson A J (1996) Evaluating neurological outcome measures: the bare essentials. Journal of Neurology, Neurosurgery and Psychiatry 60: 127–130.

Holloway R G and Dick A W (2002) Clinical trial end-points: on the road to nowhere? Neurology 58: 679–686.

Isacson O, Bjorklund L M and Schumacher J M (2003) Toward full restoration of synaptic and terminal function of the dopaminergic system in Parkinson's disease by stem cells. Annals of Neurology 53(suppl 3): S135–148.

Kim J H, Auerbach J M, Rodriguez-Gomez J A, Velasco I, Gavin D, Lumelsky N, Lee S H, Nguyen J, Sanchez-Pernaute R, Bankiewicz K and McKay R (2002) Dopamine neurons derived from embryonic stem cells function in an animal model of Parkinson's disease. Nature 418: 50–56.

Koller W C (1998) Neuroprotection for Parkinson's disease. Annals of Neurology 44(suppl 1): S155–159.

Kordower J H, Freeman T B, Snow B J, Vingerhoets F J, Mufson E J, Sanberg P R, Hauser R A, Smith D A, Nauert G M, Perl D P and Olanow C W (1995) Neuropathological evidence of graft survival and striatal reinnervation after the transplantation of fetal mesencephalic tissue in a patient with Parkinson's disease. New England Journal of Medicine 332: 1118–1124.

Kordower J H, Freeman T B, Chen E Y, Mufson E J, Sanberg P R, Hauser R A, Snow B and Olanow C W (1998) Fetal nigral grafts survive and mediate clinical benefit in a patient with Parkinson's disease. Movement Disorders 13: 383–393.

Kordower J H, Palfi S, Chen E Y, Ma SY, Sendera T, Cochran EJ, Mufson EJ, Penn R, Goetz CG, Comella CD (1999) Clinicopathological findings following intraventricular glial-derived neurotrophic factor treatment in a patient with Parkinson's disease. Annals of Neurology 46: 419–424.

Kordower J H, Emborg M E, Bloch J, Ma S Y, Chu Y, Leventhal L, McBride J, Chen E Y, Palfi S, Roitberg B Z, Brown W D, Holden J E, Pyzalski R, Taylor M D, Carvey P, Ling Z, Trono D, Hantraye P, Deglon N, Aebischer P (2000) Neurodegeneration prevented by lentiviral vector delivery of GDNF in primate models of Parkinson's disease. Science 290: 767–773.

Kukekov V G, Laywell E D, Suslov O, Davies K, Scheffler B, Thomas L B, O'Brien T F, Kusakabe M, Steindler DA (1999) Multipotent stem/progenitor cells with similar properties arise from two neurogenic regions of adult human brain. Experimental Neurology 156: 333–344.

Lang A E and Lozano A M (1998) Parkinson's disease. Second of two parts. New England Journal of Medicine 339: 1130–1143.

Lapchak P A and Araujo D M (2001) Preclinical development of trophic factors for treatment of Parkinson's disease. In: J K Krauss and J Jankovic (eds.) Surgery for Parkinson's Disease and Movement Disorders. Philadelphia: Lippincott Williams and Wilkins pp. 225–234.

Lindvall O (1994) Neural transplantation in Parkinson's disease. In: S B Dunnett and A Björklund (eds.) Functional Neural Transplantation. New York: Raven Press Ltd, pp. 103–137.

Lindvall O, Brundin P, Widner H, Rehncrona S, Gustavii B, Frackowiak R, Leenders K L, Sawle G, Rothwell J C, Marsden C D and Björklund A (1990) Grafts of fetal dopamine neurons survive and improve motor function in Parkinson's disease. Science 247: 574–577.

Lindvall O and Hagell P (2000) Clinical observations after neural transplantation in Parkinson's disease. Progress in Brain Research 27: 299–320.

Lindvall O and Hagell P (2002) Neural and stem cell transplantation. In: J Jankovic and E Tolosa (eds.) Parkinson's Disease and Movement Disorders, 4th edition. Philadelphia: Lippincott Williams and Wilkins pp. 663–673.

Ma Y, Feigin A, Dhawan V, Fukuda M, Shi Q, Greene P, Breeze R, Fahn S, Freed C and Eidelberg D (2002) Dyskinesia after fetal cell transplantation for parkinsonism: a PET study. Annals of Neurology 52: 628–634.

Mezey E, Chandross K J, Harta G, Maki R A and McKercher S R (2000) Turning blood into brain: Cells bearing neuronal antigens generated in vivo from bone marrow. Science 290: 1779–1782.

Morrish P (2002) Is it time to abandon functional imaging in the study of neuroprotection? Movement Disorders 17: 229–232.

Morrish P (2003) REAL and CALM: What have we learned? Movement Disorders 18: 839–840.

Mytilineou C, Radcliffe P M and Olanow C W (1997) L-(-)-desmethylselegiline, a metabolite of selegiline [L-(-)-deprenyl], protects mesencephalic dopamine neurons from excitotoxicity in vitro. Journal of Neurochemistry 68: 434–436.

Nutt J G, Burchiel K J, Comella C L, Jankovic J, Lang A E, Laws E R Jr, Lozano A M, Penn R D, Simpson R K Jr, Stacy M, Wooten G F and ICV GDNF Study Group (2003) Randomized, double-blind trial of glial cell line-derived neurotrophic factor (GDNF) in PD. Neurology 60:69–73.

Obinu M C, Reibaud M, Blanchard V, Moussaoui S and Imperato A (2002) Neuroprotective effect of riluzole in a primate model of Parkinson's disease: behavioral and histological evidence. Movement Disorders 17: 13–19.

Ohta M, Mizuta I, Ohta K, Nishimura M, Mizuta E, Hayashi K and Kuno S (2000) Apomorphine upregulates NGF and GDNF synthesis in cultured mouse astrocytes. Biochemical and Biophysical Research Communications 272: 18–22.

Olanow C W, Jenner P and Brooks D J (1998) Dopamine agonists and neuroprotection in Parkinson's disease. Annals of Neurology 44(suppl 1): S167–174.

Olanow C W, Watts R L and Koller W C (2001) An algorithm (decision tree) for the management of Parkinson's disease (2001): treatment guidelines. Neurology 56(Suppl 5): S1–88.

Olanow C W, Goetz C G, Kordower J H, Stoessl A J, Sossi V, Brin M F, Shannon K M, Nauert G M, Perl D P, Godbold J and Freeman T B (2003) A double-blind controlled trial of bilateral fetal nigral transplantation in Parkinson's disease. Annals of Neurology 54: 403–414.

Parkinson Study Group (1989) Effect of deprenyl on the progression of disability in early Parkinson's disease. New England Journal of Medicine 321: 1364–1371.

Parkinson Study Group (2002) Dopamine transporter brain imaging to assess the effects of pramipexole vs levodopa on Parkinson disease progression. Journal of the American Medical Association 287: 1653–1661.

Piallat B, Benazzouz A and Benabid A L (1999) Neuroprotective effect of chronic inactivation of the subthalamic nucleus in a rat model of Parkinson's disease. Journal of Neural Transmission 55(suppl): 71–77.

Piccini P, Brooks D J, Björklund A, Gunn R N, Grasby P M, Rimoldi O, Brundin P, Hagell P, Rehncrona S, Widner H and Lindvall O (1999) Dopamine release from nigral transplants visualized in vivo in a Parkinson's patient. Nature Neuroscience 2: 1137–1140.

Piccini P, Lindvall O, Björklund A, Brundin P, Hagell P, Ceravolo R, Oertel W, Quinn N, Samuel M, Rehncrona S, Widner H and Brooks D J (2000) Delayed recovery of movement–related cortical function in Parkinson's disease after striatal dopaminergic grafts. Annals of Neurology 48: 689–695.

Quinn N P (1998) Classification of fluctuations in patients with Parkinson's disease. Neurology 51(suppl 2): S25–29.

Rascol O, Olanow W, Brooks D, et al (2002) A 2-year, multicenter, placebo-controlled, double-blind, parallel-group study of the effect of riluzole on Parkinson's disease progression. Movement Disorders 17(suppl 5): S39.

Rodriguez M C, Obeso J A and Olanow C W (1998) Subthalamic nucleus-mediated excitotoxicity in Parkinson's disease: A target for neuroprotection. Annals of Neurology 44(suppl 1): S175–188.

Scheife R T, Schumock G T, Burstein A, Gottwald M D and Luer M S (2000) Impact of Parkinson's disease and its pharmacologic treatment on quality of life and economic outcomes. American Journal of Health-System Pharmacy 57: 953–962.

Shoulson I and the Parkinson Study Group (1998) DATATOP: A decade of neuroprotective inquiry. Annals of Neurology 44(suppl 1): S160–166.

Siderowf A, Holloway R and Mushlin A (1998) Cost-effectiveness of pallidotomy and add-on medical therapy in Parkinson's disease. Annals of Neurology 44: 517.

Steindler D A and Pincus D W (2002) Stem cells and neuropoiesis in the adult human brain. Lancet 359: 1047–1054.

Stross R, Mallon G, O'Sullivan K, Joint C (2004) A practical guide to deep brain stimulation and other movement disorders. PDNSA.

Studer L, Tabar V and McKay R D (1998) Transplantation of expanded mesencephalic precursors leads to recovery in parkinsonian rats. Nature Neuroscience 1: 290–295.

Tatton W G and Greenwood C E (1991) Rescue of dying neurons: a new action for deprenyl in MPTP parkinsonism. Journal of Neuroscience Research 30: 666–672.

Tenenbaum L, Chtarto A, Lehtonen E, Blum D, Baekelandt V, Velu T, Brotchi J and Levivier M. (2002) Neuroprotective gene therapy for Parkinson's disease. Current Gene Therapy 2: 451–483.

Tetrud J W and Langston J W (1989) The effect of deprenyl (selegiline) on the natural history of Parkinson's disease. Science 245: 519–522.

Ying Q L, Nichols J, Evans E P and Smith A G (2002) Changing potency by spontaneous fusion. Nature 416; 545–548.

Whone A L, Watts R L, Stoessl A J, Davis M, Reske S, Nahmias C, Lang A E, Rascol O, Ribeiro M J, Remy P, Poewe W H, Hauser R A, Brooks D J and REAL-PET Study Group. (2003) Slower progression of Parkinson's disease treated with ropinirole versus levodopa: the REAL-PET study. Annals of Neurology 54: 93–101.

Wright B D (1997) Fundamental measurement for outcome evaluation. Physical Medicine and Rehabilitation: State of the Art Reviews 11: 261–288.

Index

Note The following abbreviations are used in the index: DBS (deep brain stimulation), MSA (multiple system atrophy), PD (Parkinson's disease) and PSP (progressive supranuclear palsy).